Dr Sigrid Flade

GW00692335

# Natural remedies for allergies

- help for sufferers of hay fever, asthma, eczema, food allergies and their after-effects
- tests and methods of treatment
- directions for self-help

TIME-LIFE BOOKS, AMSTERDAM

## Important Note

The views expressed by the authors of the HEALTH CARE TODAY series may differ in part from generally recognized orthodox medicine. All readers must decide for themselves whether, and to what extent, they wish to follow the advice given in this book. It is important to stress that seemingly mild ailments may occasionally conceal serious illnesses which must be treated by a qualified medical practitioner. If in doubt, you should seek expert medical advice at the earliest opportunity. Every form of therapy has its limitations and these must be respected.

*Dedicated to my son, Uli*

# Contents

# Contents

# Foreword

Allergies are on the increase! Doctors are reporting that more and more patients are coming to them for advice about hay fever, asthma, nettle rash, eczema or contact dermatitis. In fact, you probably wouldn't have picked up this book unless you, or someone close to you, is suffering from an allergy of some kind.

As well as known allergies, there are a large number that still remain undiagnosed. For example, food allergies which may present a variety of symptoms such as disorientation, exhaustion, drowsiness, lack of concentration, irritability, hyperactivity, headaches, migraine, dizziness, depression, irregular heartbeat, excess weight, constipation, diarrhoea or rheumatic joint complaints, are often hard to identify.

Even though allergies are on the increase, it would seem that this is one area where conventional medicine has few effective weapons at its disposal for bringing about a complete cure. Many dissatisfied patients, in their search for help, are now turning to 'alternative' therapies.

I strongly believe that doctors should not leave their patients to go down the alternative route alone. This is why, after nearly 25 years of orthodox medical work in a large clinic, I decided to study natural medicine to find out how it worked and if it could help allergy sufferers.

I was astonished by what I discovered: a whole branch of medicine has grown out of the age-old tradition of naturopathy. And it has done this not least through incorporating modern technology, based on the latest biophysical discoveries.

Because of the number and variety of the methods and therapies used, alternative medicine can be complex and multi-layered so that years of intensive study are required in order to gain a complete mastery of the subject and the various techniques. However, some of the basic techniques are simple and can be used easily at home.

To understand natural medicine we have to reconsider the nature of illness and of healing. This, and treatment methods that are not yet common knowledge, form the subject matter of this book.

Every doctor learns from his or her own experience and

the path to success is different for each person. So there is an unavoidable degree of subjectiveness in both my views and advice on therapies, medicines and their sources.

My main aim is to discover ways in which the alarming increase in allergy-related illnesses can be countered. I see this as a task that calls for a joint effort from all of us:

● doctors, by incorporating the theory and practice of natural medicine into therapeutic procedures more extensively than at present;

● the National Health Service and private medical insurers, by accepting the costs of such treatment;

● patients, by taking responsibility for their own health;

● and all of us, by fighting the threat to our health and existence that is posed by the pollution of our environment – the background against which this increase in allergies must be viewed.

I owe a debt of gratitude to all those colleagues I've had the opportunity of learning from and who, over past decades and in spite of a great amount of hostility, have unwaveringly conserved and expanded the knowledge and added to the treasury of empirical natural healing methods.

My thanks must also go to Carl Hermann Ebbinghaus for all the support he has given me along the way, not least for his expert and knowledgeable revision of the manuscript of this book.

*Dr Sigrid Flade*

# Learn to think in a different way

Allergies
and the
environment

Allergies are not like ordinary illnesses where medicine can be used to treat the cause. Allergies occur as a direct result of the way people live and their environment, and the things that cause them cannot be cured by medicine. The great increase in allergy-related illnesses is now forcing people to acknowledge that the industrial age they are living in is developing in a way that threatens both their health and well-being.

If you suffer from an allergy it is likely that it is caused by modern living. This means that to avoid allergies you will need to make some serious changes to the way you live.

Until recently people's lifestyles have been influenced by the incredible technical advances that have taken place this century. Many of these advances have helped to ease workloads and give people an easier, more comfortable life. But the destruction this new technical age is causing to the environment has gradually forced people to realize that it is endangering not only their own health, but also that of their children and grandchildren.

If we want to work towards saving the environment we will have to rethink our values and make substantial changes to the way we live. To begin with we need to rid ourselves of any superficial notions of progress and be prepared, in whole areas of our everyday lives, to rethink the way we do things.

Consider
and act

This is not a simple thing to do, especially when we consider how much easier life has become through technological progress. Although people can be both inventive and adaptable in times of need and scarcity, in prosperous times they often think only of themselves and the satisfaction of their immediate desires. Their time is spent in pursuit of the maximum possible pleasure, with much of their thinking governed by things such as when they are going to buy a new car or a second television set.

Today people are gradually waking up to the damage that is being done to the environment and are becoming less at ease with their current lifestyle. But, even so, many continue with their old habits and carry on living improvidently from one day to the next.

**We are all responsible**

You may feel that governments are not doing enough to help the environment. But recent worldwide concern indicates that there is a growing awareness amongst the world's nations of the problems we are all facing. New laws and regulations are not necessarily the long-term answer. In the end we are all responsible. We have to be prepared to assume responsibility for ourselves, in both our work and home environments, and to take joint responsibility for the world at large.

This means getting used to thinking ahead and being aware. For example, did you know that the propellant gas that was used in aerosols was partly responsible for the hole in the ozone layer that surrounds the earth? As this hole becomes bigger it will eventually lead to an increased risk of cancer, as well as climatic changes which will have an enormous impact on the environment.

Even knowing this, it is all too easy to pay more attention to the present – how your hair looks for a night out at the theatre – than to any natural disasters that may be expected to occur in the distant future.

**Think about the effects of your actions**

People don't normally think about the consequences of actions that won't come to light until some time in the future, even if these actions do affect the entire human race. But this kind of thoughtlessness could, in the long term, cost you, your children and grandchildren everything.

What is happening to the environment is seen by many people as one of the most threatening situations in the history of the earth. However, you can find hope in the fact that there are more and more people who are beginning to recognize the signs and are showing awareness of the dangers. These people are prepared to stand up for the environment, make sacrifices for it and will try to influence others to join them. They have assumed responsibility for their own health and will find out for themselves the best way to maintain it, and to combat the stresses and strains of daily life.

A radically different line of thought is gaining acceptance in all classes of society and amongst all age groups. People who follow it recognize that humanity is part of a whole.

**Mankind is part of nature**   They see themselves as an integral part of nature, subject to its laws, and recognize that they shouldn't do things without any thought, just because they are technically possible.

This type of thinking shows the sharp contrast between people who are trying to counter impending dangers, and those who simply close their eyes to them.

### Orthodox medicine – and natural medicine

Such contradictory attitudes can be observed wherever conclusions have to be drawn from changed circumstances. Naturally, this is also true of medicine.

People have been lulled by decades of unprecedented medical progress into a belief that practically anything is possible. Vaccines and a steady flow of new antibiotics have freed people from the dangers of infectious diseases, which in the past killed so many in their prime. Painkillers, sleeping pills and rheumatism pills make it easier to bear illness. Replacement surgery copes with the loss of teeth, a leg, a hip, even a kidney. This kind of progressive development is opening up new possibilities in intensive medicine, anaesthesia and surgical techniques.

For many, their doctor is considered the expert in all matters relating to health so that they take, without asking too many questions, whatever is prescribed for them. The view often expressed is that it is up to the doctor to make them healthy again, and it's up to the NHS to pay the bill.

But these days patients, doctors and the NHS are having to lower their expectations of what modern science can achieve. More and more patients are becoming dissatisfied with the results of conventional medicine. They are finding that they only get temporary alleviation of symptoms, but they are not actually being cured.   **The critical patient**

Consequently more and more people are turning to natural treatment methods and, increasingly, are also prepared to do something about their own health, such as changing over to a diet which includes wholefoods, taking more exercise and giving up smoking.

Doctors, too, are having to face up to the fact that, despite advances in research, there are limits to what modern medicine can achieve. This is especially true in the case of chronic illnesses where sophisticated techniques are used for diagnosis, but the treatments available do not usually lead to a complete cure.

This is why some doctors have already turned to natural medicine as a means of treating chronic illnesses. But for a great number of doctors there are practical difficulties involved in doing this. Although there are an increasing number of courses, seminars and congresses about natural medicine on offer, to study the subject in the depth required to be able to practise it, takes a great deal of time. Because of their already heavy workload, some doctors feel that they are not able to find the additional time that would be required for this.

**The committed doctor**

However, those that have become involved in natural medicine are usually great proponents of it. Their enthusiasm has made other health care professionals rethink their attitude to this type of medicine. This rethinking process has gradually begun to spread to the NHS and to some, far-sighted, health insurance companies. Until recently insurance companies have refused to cover payments for any form of natural healing because the effect of the treatment could not be explained scientifically. Now, in view of the number of patients who have been treated successfully, some insurance companies have become more open-minded about natural medicine. This attitude may have been helped by the fact that medical costs could rise to prohibitive levels in the future unless treatments, which lead to complete cures are found.

**Health insurance companies become more open-minded**

# The paths to healing

Instead of
fighting
symptoms
with
chemicals...
There is an enormous number of medicines available both on prescription or over-the-counter at the pharmacy. Many of these are produced to combat everyday complaints such as coughs, colds, fever, diarrhoea, pain and inflammation. What many people do not realize is that these symptoms are usually a sign that our body is calling on its natural healing powers as it tries to fight off an illness. For example, it has been scientifically proven that during a fever the high temperature will kill off viruses and help to activate the body's own defence system. So, when we take medicine to suppress symptoms, we interfere with the body's natural healing process.

Natural medicine aims to strengthen and support the body's healing processes by natural means, such as compresses, baths, diet and homeopathic medicines. It is used for chronic diseases, rheumatism, allergies and a susceptibility to infection and boils. It works by harmonizing the body's functions and strengthening the immune system so that, with the support of a wholefood diet rich in minerals and vitamins, it is possible to achieve a noticeable change for the better.

... support
your own
powers of
self-healing

By using natural medicine you can overcome illness by bringing the body into peak condition without subjecting it to the stress of chemical agents (which almost always have side-effects).

Of course, this doesn't mean that conventional medicine becomes superfluous. Antibiotics are still needed to cure some infections; in primary chronic polyarthritis the appropriate rheumatism pills help to ensure freedom from pain; insulin, essential for the treatment of diabetes, has to be replaced artificially, and cortisone is needed to counteract serious allergic reactions.

A doctor has to find the right treatment for each individual patient, based on what they themselves are like as well as their illness. This means that the doctor, in addition to his knowledge of orthodox medicine, also needs to have a detailed understanding of natural medicine. It is also important that the patient has some understanding of how the healing process works.

**Patients play an active role**

Where once a patient's cooperation in the healing process was confined to taking a particular medicine three times a day, it's an absolute precondition of natural medicine that the patient plays an active role. Working together with the doctor as a partner, the patient assumes responsibility for his own health.

# How do allergic reactions begin?

When allergens, such as pollen, animal hairs, house dust and certain foods enter the body they are recognized by the blood cells that form part of the body's immune system. These cells then produce antibodies which are specific to the allergen. The antibodies attach themselves to cells in the tissues called mast cells. These mast cells contain a substance called histamine. Allergens bind to the antibodies on the surface of the mast cells and this leads to the release of histamine and to the symptoms of allergy.

The skin and mucous membranes react by becoming red and swollen and this is often accompanied by excessive secretions. This may lead to an attack of hay fever, asthma, nettle rash or even diarrhoea

**Allergy means an exaggerated reaction of the immune system**

In orthodox medicine, this classic sequence at the start of an illness is what is meant by the term 'allergy' – an exaggerated reaction of the immune system to a variety of substances.

It is important to distinguish allergies from intolerance or sensitivity. These also cause a discharge of histamine and occur as a result of sensitivity to chemical additives or impurities in food, for example, colourants, preservatives, antifungal agents, pesticide residues, sorbic acid, benzoic acid, sulphites in dried fruits, wines and ready-to-eat potato products, and some medicines, such as aspirin. Their effect on the patient is the same as the symptoms of allergy so it is easy to confuse the two.

## Testing methods

There are two types of tests used to diagnose the cause of an allergy – skin tests and blood tests. These procedures are not foolproof but they can help to identify the cause of an allergy. The best match is obtained for pollen, dust and other airborne allergens. Skin tests involving animal hairs, fungi and mites are more accurate than those used to diagnose food allergies which are known to be particularly unreliable. Skin tests are simple to perform and cause only a minimal amount of discomfort. Blood tests may cause some discomfort and are often rather less sensitive than the skin tests.

**Tests are not foolproof**

## Skin tests

**Scratch test:** The surface of the skin is scratched on the inner side of the lower arm and the appropriate test extracts are applied.

**Prick test:** A drop of a particular allergen solution is applied to the skin on the inside of the lower arm. The surface of the skin is then pricked with a needle. After 15-30 minutes the reaction is noted.

**Intradermal test:** A small amount of sterile allergen solution is injected into the skin on the inner side of the lower arm.

**Rubbing test:** The skin of the lower arm is firmly rubbed eight to ten times with the allergen (animal hairs, egg-white, fish, vegetables, dust). If there is an allergic reaction, prominences the size of a pinhead will appear after two to three minutes and grow into larger spots within 20 minutes.

**Mucous-membrane test:** The allergen is applied to the conjunctiva, or the mucous membrane of the nasal cavity (in the bronchial provocation test, it is inhaled), and the patient is observed for symptoms.

**Linen-patch test:** The test substances in either the form of drops or ointment are placed on small linen patches which are then stuck to the skin of the back. The test usually takes between 48 and 72 hours to complete.

## Blood tests

**RAST** (radioallergosorbent test) and (chemoluminescence assay) are used to show the presence of individual allergens.

**Cyto** (cytotoxological test) detects food allergies. This test, developed in the USA, is not yet a routine procedure here. Its advantage is its wide range: it tests 181 different foods.

It is important to note that none of these testing methods is completely reliable.

# What triggers allergies?

The potential triggers for allergic illnesses can be found in a surprisingly large range of substances, both natural and synthetic. In every case an allergy is sparked off by a quite specific set of allergens so, if you could avoid these you would not be affected by the allergy. However, this is rarely possible, or indeed practical, so the best we can usually hope to achieve is a reduction in the amount of the allergen in our environment so that we can obtain some relief from the organism.

**Allergens in your environment** Laboratory tests may be able to pinpoint specific substances which cause an allergic reaction, but you can discover a lot from self-observation. Once allergens are diagnosed you should try to minimize their level in your own environment to reduce their effect. This is something that no doctor can do for you.

By becoming an active partner in your own recovery you can go a long way towards removing the need for regular long-term medication. For example, if you suffer from asthma you need to work hard at removing the mites from your bed or the fungi from the walls, and you may have to get rid of any furniture made with formaldehyde products, such as some foams.

It is important to know how an allergy can be triggered, or made to persist. Once you have discovered this you need to consider whether you have done enough to remove the allergens from your own environment.

## Fungi

Allergy to fungi is becoming increasingly frequent nowadays. Fungal spores are inhaled, and the allergen they contain causes a discharge of histamine in the antibodies of the bronchial mucous membrane. This can result in coughing, mucous congestion and breathing difficulties.

Fungi grow wherever there is damp, dirt or rotting materials such as leaves, earth or refuse. In buildings, they can be found on windows, pot plants, damp walls and wallpaper, in beds and mattresses, cellars and attics. Swimming pools, greenhouses, bathrooms and animal stalls

**Fungal spores are everywhere**

are favourite breeding places for fungi. Air conditioning units and humidifiers help to spread them throughout the atmosphere.

Given away by mildew

You will also find fungi where there is mildew, and this can be found almost anywhere in the home, even on leather shoes and furniture.

Fungi prosper especially well when the humidity is around 80 per cent and the average temperature is 20°C. So, if your asthma gets worse in warm, damp weather or in the autumn, when there are rotting leaves about, there is good reason to suspect fungal allergy.

Different species of fungi release their spores at different times over several months – some around noon, others in the evening, at night or in the morning. The greatest number of spores are released in February, March, August and September.

It is not always possible to see fungi. Food, fresh fruit juice and alcoholic beverages such as wine, beer or champagne, can be contaminated by fungi without showing any immediately visible signs. Foods to watch out for are: fruit and vegetables, dried fruits, black pepper, nuts, cereals such as muesli, cheese, yeast and sauerkraut.

**Fungi can be invisible**

Anyone who finds it difficult to tolerate a particular type of fruit or vegetable will need to consider the possibility that they have a fungal allergy rather than just an intolerance to that food.

Enzymes, some of which are a refined fungal product, are used in large quantities in the manufacture of foodstuffs as well as many other everyday products. These include common household items such as leather, soap, detergents (especially biological ones), cosmetics, bath products and even toothpastes.

If you find that any of these affect you, or that a particular medicine, for example penicillin (which is made from a fungus) causes an allergic reaction, you may want to consider the possibility that you are suffering from an allergy to fungi.

You may
only need to
do some of
these things
to get better

## How to combat fungi

● First of all, the breeding area of the fungus must be cleaned as thoroughly as possible. Damp walls must be dried out and mouldy areas replastered. If you use an air conditioning unit have it regularly checked and cleaned.

● You can buy products that will kill fungi at the chemist, but it is likely that many of these will contain dangerous chemicals.

● Get rid of any houseplants as these can often be a breeding ground for fungi. You will also need to do without humidifiers and atomizers.

● Wash fruit and vegetables with particular care. Peel fruit whenever possible.

● Try to avoid all manufactured products that may contain fungal enzymes.

● Use alternatives such as calcium carbonate, which you can buy at the chemist, to take the place of toothpaste, and soap flakes or natural soap instead of biological detergents. Ask the manufacturer to give you a list of ingredients of any products that you are unsure about.

Find
alternatives

● Avoid animal stalls, zoos and greenhouses, and don't walk in the woods in autumn.

As a rule, fungal allergies occur in combination with allergies to house dust, mites, pollen and foods.

## Mites

You may feel certain that you have no creepy-crawlies in your clean, well cared for home, and you may be offended if anyone said otherwise. But you would be wrong!

Mites are
secret
lodgers

In Europe mites are secret lodgers in every dwelling. They like to make their nests in mattresses, bedclothes, cushions, carpets and cuddly toys. A room temperature of 15-30°C (25°C for preference) and humidity of 55-85 per cent (ideally 75 per cent) make favourable conditions for the development of mites. Mites multiply most feverishly between May and October but they can survive the bad times in the form of larvae or eggs, to reproduce once more when conditions improve. The allergen isn't the mite itself but its excrement. This is produced in growing measure during the summer months, so complaints increase correspondingly in the autumn.

**The allergens in the excrement**

You will get an indication that you're suffering from a mite allergy if, for example, you suffer acute discomfort when using a vacuum cleaner. Symptoms may worsen when you're going to bed, getting up or making the bed, because mites prefer to sit at the top and bottom of the bedclothes and are shaken up at such times.

These parasites have a particularly comfortable time in your bed: your body heat and the moisture you exude create an ideal breeding climate. These favourable conditions for the mites are maintained if, on getting up, you cover the bed again straight away instead of letting it air thoroughly. Another plus point for mites is that their main nourishment is delivered on the spot, in the shape of the flakes of skin shed continually by your body.

### How to combat mites

- Get rid of old mattresses, cushions and upholstered furniture.

**Vacuum thoroughly**

- Vacuum very thoroughly. Experiments have shown that, even after a full minute of vacuuming, only eight per cent of the mites in any square metre are eliminated. Amazingly, only if the same square metre is vacuumed more than 40 times a day, for at least four consecutive days, can the majority of the mites and their excrement be eliminated.
- Use one of the preparations that are available for killing mites. You can buy these from the chemist in foam or powder form. You can successfully treat fitted carpets, mattresses and bedclothes this way.

Remember that, as these are chemical preparations, you should check before using them (by sniffing) to see whether they cause you any problems themselves.

## House dust

Mite allergy, like fungal allergy, can't be separated from house-dust allergy, because mite excrement and fungal spores spread along with the dust.

Generally, house dust has a wide variety of ingredients: tiny particles of dirt and rust from the air, wood fibres, bedding feathers, hair and, most of all, flakes of skin from humans and animals.

**Mixing of allergens**

### Helping yourself

**Protect yourself from house dust**

● Avoid all dust-traps in your home. Dust mostly gathers in carpets and carpeting, so floors that you can mop are better.
● Keep your books in enclosed bookcases rather than on open shelves, and don't keep books in your bedroom.
● Avoid fitting embossed or textured carpets as they are real dust-traps.
● Wipe dust away with a damp cloth to avoid raising clouds of it. Don't forget the radiators, dust from which is carried into the room by rising warm air.
● To prevent dusty air being blown out of your vacuum cleaner, use special filters or water tanks (a central vacuuming plant is even better). You can also set up ionizers to remove dust and pollen from the air.

## Animals

Hairs and flakes of skin from animals, not to mention their excrement and saliva, are frequent allergens. This applies especially to pets such as dogs, cats, horses, rabbits, guinea pigs, hamsters and birds.

**Pets can cause allergies**

Although children learn a lot from having a pet to love and care for, pets can cause serious problems for anyone in the family suffering from an allergy. Sometimes an allergy is not detected until sometime after the arrival of a pet, which makes it hard for everyone concerned as often the only answer is for the pet to be rehoused elsewhere.

Being told that the only solution is to get rid of a much-loved animal often meets with resistance, especially if the allergy to the pet is not obvious. But this lack of a direct link is normal when an allergy sufferer lives in the constant company of an animal. The allergy is latent in this case, so a direct link with the symptoms is no more evident than, for example, a wheat allergy when bread is eaten daily.

**Latent allergy**

You can put it to the test by sending your pet away from home for a while and then thoroughly vacuuming and cleaning up. If symptoms are alleviated during this period, only to worsen on your pet's return, then there's good chance that the pet is causing the allergy. If the results are otherwise, it could be that other allergens remaining in the home (such as mites or fungi) are preventing any improvement.

There are different degrees of animal-hair allergy: in minor cases, symptoms occur only when the animal is moulting heavily. With a serious allergy, however, the sufferer reacts with cold symptoms, asthma, coughing or eczema, even if he just meets someone who keeps a pet. Small quantities of animal hair or flakes of skin on clothing are enough to trigger such reactions.

**Animal-hair allergy**

No allergy need be feared in the case of fish, but fish food can cause strong reactions. A tortoise is almost always allergen free, but you need to make sure that dust, fungi and mites don't accumulate in the place where it lives.

### How to protect yourself from animal allergies

● Avoid homes where there are pets and keep away from animal stalls and zoos.

● If you have a pet and you think it may be causing the allergy give it to someone else to look after for a few weeks to see whether not having it around makes a difference. If the pet is causing the allergy you may need to consider finding it a new home.

● Avoid all animal products such as wool, fur and even leather in your clothes and furniture. This may sound surprising, as a common belief is that 'natural' materials must be healthier than anything artificial and synthetic. For allergy sufferers, however, this is not necessarily always the case.

**Avoid animal products**

# Pollen

Allergy to pollen, the male germ cells of flowering plants, is a widespread affliction. It causes hay fever – which is by no means confined to hay – and asthma. Pollen allergy can also intensify eczema.

**Germ cells of flowering plants**

Pollen grains contain more than 12 different substances to which allergic people often over-react. Normally, each of us inhales 4,000-5,000 pollen grains every day without our bodies showing any sign of being affected by them. But for people with an allergy 40-50 pollen grains are often enough to set off an allergic reaction.

A wide range of pollens from flowers, grasses, trees and weeds cause allergies, and every sufferer has his own specific allergen pattern.

**Pollen calendar**

A large number of plants flower from February to April. These include: hazel, poplar, birch, alder, willow, beech and elm. Anyone who reacts to these may also, under some circumstances, show incompatibility with apples, pears, cherries, gooseberries, blackcurrants, peaches and grapes.

Anyone who suffers from a dripping nose from May to July, or whose allergic rections last until September, is probably suffering from an allergy to the pollen of grass or cereals, or is allergic to new-mown grass or hay. If the latter applies it is best to leave mowing the lawn to a non-suffering relative and avoid trips through the countryside in the hay-making season.

If you suffer in August and September, you may have an allergy to weeds, particularly plantain and mugwort. This is often combined with an allergy to various herbs such as dill, caraway, pepper, nutmeg, paprika, parsley, mustard or cinnamon.

## Limited protection from pollen

● Radio and TV stations broadcast pollen warnings so that you can tell from day to day what the risk is of suffering an

**Take heed of pollen warnings**

attack of hay fever or asthma. There is also a number of telephone helplines which carry similar information so it is worth checking these as well.

● You can only protect yourself up to a point. Since pollen begins to take to the air at around four in the morning, you'll need to have your bedroom window closed before then. The greatest concentration of pollen in the air occurs at around midday. In hot summer weather, however, pollen can rise so high that it doesn't cause symptoms until the evening, when the cooling air brings it back down to earth. Other than that you can only hope for rain, which brings relief to most hay fever sufferers. Or you could furnish a room in the cellar, and move in there when the torment becomes too much to bear!

● Remember the flowering season when planning your holiday: in the south, spring can come quite a few weeks earlier than in the north.

Your hay fever may explode with particular violence if you treat yourself to an Easter holiday in southern climes. This is likely to expose you to a sudden bombardment of pollen that your body will not be able to withstand. So you need to think carefully about your holiday destination. You may find that you have a far better time somewhere like the Isle of Skye, or in the mountains, preferably above the deciduous tree line, or in an area where there are no flowering plants, such as a Greek island in summer.

**Plan your holiday carefully**

# Harbingers of allergy

## Amalgam

There is far too little awareness of the possibility that the metals contained in dental amalgam can harm your health, especially if there is another metal in your mouth such as a gold inlay, a metal bridge or a brace. A weak, galvanic electric current can flow within your mouth, causing the mercury ions to be dissolved out of the fillings, and then travel via the jaw tissue and the lymph channels into the intestines, the kidneys, the liver and, worst of all, the brain.

A wide range of symptoms can be triggered in this way: restless sleep, inability to concentrate, poor memory, nervousness, trembling, depressions, dizziness, migraine, cardiovascular disturbances and circulatory disorders.

It's important for allergy sufferers to know that asthma, eczema and even food allergies, with their variety of symptoms, can be triggered off by dental amalgam.

Naturally, most people suffer no apparent harm from the amalgam fillings in their teeth. But the number of those whose health is damaged, sometimes extremely seriously, by their fillings and who traipse from doctor to doctor in search of a cure, is higher than was originally supposed.

Mercury poisoning from amalgam fillings can often be a harbinger of an allergic reaction. Investigations using blood tests, as well as some specialist electro-acupuncture techniques can help identify mercury problems. If necessary, amalgam fillings may have to be replaced with gold, or a similarly non-allergic, synthetic material.

Palladium, a metal which is a component in some gold inlays, can also cause reactions similar to amalgam fillings. If your crowns or inlays contain palladium, then take an electro-acupuncture test to find out if there is a problem.

**Mercury poisoning from your fillings**

## Domestic poisons

People who suffer from eczema and asthma, often find that even intensive biological treatment is ineffective if there are poisons in the home which continue to aggravate the illness. The chief offenders here are formaldehyde and wood preservatives.

**Formaldehyde:** contained in cosmetics, creams, shampoos, felt-tipped pens and, in particular, in furniture made of foam or chipboard (frequently used for cupboards and cheap children's furniture), in sealed parquet flooring and glued carpets. Even when you can no longer smell the formaldehyde it still continues to be dangerous, as it can continue to give off gases which can damage your health for up to 20 years.

Anyone who has become sensitized to this material may react to even the smallest quantities of it. Young children and people with a tendency to allergies are in particular danger. Typical symptoms include burning and watering eyes, throat inflammations, chronic coughing, headaches, dizziness, vomiting, sleeplessness, nervousness, memory loss, depression, poor concentration, and a variety of other painful conditions, including circulatory and cardiovascular problems.

If the delicate mucous membranes in your nose and throat are damaged, pathogenic organisms can establish themselves more easily, and then permanent cold symptoms and sinusitis can ensue. The development of sensitivity to fungi, pollen, house dust or food gives allergies a boost.

Formaldehyde has been classified as a carcinogen, in other words a cancer-causing substance, by the European Community. Exposure to formaldehyde can be detected from a urine sample and formaldehyde in the air can also be measured with specialist equipment.

You will need to contact a specialist group to find out more about these particular tests. They should also be able to help if you want to have a formaldehyde test carried out.

**Wood preservatives:** like formaldehyde, lindane and pentachlorophenol can have a disastrous effect on your health. Anyone handling wood in and around the home

*Harmful substances can give off gases for up to 20 years*

*Typical symptoms*

needs to be aware of the possible risks from wood preservatives. Your health could be damaged for life just through handling wooden floorboards, wooden interior beams, window and door openings, or even an old-fashioned wooden cupboard. Tests on materials such as house dust, samples of carpet or timber can be made to see if the interior of a building is contaminated with lindane or pentachlorophenol. A blood or urine test will provide more information.

**Avoidable health risk**

**Tests can be carried out**

**Pesticides:** allergy sufferers need to be selective when buying fresh fruit and vegetables. Only organically grown produce is guaranteed to be free from chemical fertilizers and pesticides. It is not only the pesticide residues in the food that help to cause allergies, but also the substances sprayed on the crops as they are growing. In extreme cases people with asthma have found that the 'healthy country air' causes them more problems than the pollution of the city. Organophosphates used in sheep dip may also cause similar problems.

**Buy only unsprayed fruit**

## Terrestrial and cosmic radiation

People are exposed not just to cosmic, but also to terrestrial radiation – rays that come from deep below the surface of of the earth. This radiation does not necessarily emerge uniformly from the earth but can be amplified in bands, via electrically-conductive objects in the underlying rock, such as rift and fault zones, chasms, underground waterways (water veins), and sometimes via seams of coal, oil or ore, or conductive rock.

**Rays from the depths of the earth**

Therapies are often not completely successful, even where allergies are concerned, as long as the patient continues to sleep in an unhealthy bedroom.

In Europe, the most significant feature is underground waterways (particularly their intersections at various depths) and faults or geological rift zones that cause areas of disturbance or irritation.

Terrestrial radiation can penetrate even the thickest layers of iron and concrete. The strength of the radiation does not diminish with height. Its intensity is as great on the top storey of a skyscraper as it is on the surface of the earth. The radiation can even continue to build up a charge via the steel reinforcement in concrete buildings. These narrowly confine this terrestrial radiation, which is then restricted into a narrow vertical channel.

**Radiation from the cosmos**

But that isn't all. There are further geometrical strip systems that aren't affected by the geology underneath the surface. As far as is known at present, these are the consequences of standing electromagnetic waves originating from space, which are guided by the earth's magnetic field. These waves of radiation are variously known as Dr Hartmann's global grid, Dr Curry's network, and also as the Benker grid.

A special strain is imposed on our bodies where these grid areas coincide with terrestrial disturbances, for example with an underground water vein or an intersection between veins of water. These 'radiation' problems are often described as geopathic stress.

If you suffer from frequent complaints this may be because your bed is positioned at a place of disturbance.

You should consider this if you:
- take hours to get to sleep
- don't sleep peacefully
- rumple your bedclothes
- have nightmares
- call out in your sleep
- sleepwalk
- grind your teeth or feel them chattering
- experience sweating or freezing spells at night
- fall out of bed
- or if children roll over in their sleep to one side, or to the foot of the bed, or wake up crying.

The consequences the day after such a bad night include extreme tiredness, which often lasts throughout the day. This may be accompanied by feelings of nervousness and depression, cramps, palpitations, migraine and even bouts of aggression.

The unhealthy effect of such radiation has long been known to ancient cultures such as the Chinese, Celts and African medicine men. Buildings, such as the pyramids were erected on previously undisturbed sites that had been checked with a divining rod (a forked hazel twig).

**Checking with a divining rod**

Water was found in the same way. Water authorities still occasionally use a dowser's services. The human senses that can detect such weak energy levels are also used when a bedroom or perhaps a building site has to be checked.

This requires a certain talent, which about half the population has, a thorough knowledge of the technique and stable health. Nowadays, divining rods are made from bent welding rods, brass or plastic.

The dowser takes up a position near, say, a water vein. If he gets closer to it, his nerve centre reacts by causing muscular tensions which are transmitted to the rod and make it swing up or down.

All of this may sound like pure hocus-pocus. But you need to remember that our bodies are controlled by the most subtle energies, which they can register with corresponding sensitivity. The first steps have already been taken towards objective measurement using VHF and the body's intrinsic resistance.

Already some governments have commissioned research studies into subjects such as 'the human perception of terrestrial radiation'. This could be seen as a sign that the possibility of damage to health from terrestrial radiation is being taken seriously by official bodies.

**Sensitivity to negative influences during sleep**

There is an argument that says that people are not aware of anything in their sleep. But we are in fact particularly sensitive during sleep to negative influences on our environment. Besides terrestrial radiation, these include a whole series of disturbing factors that we now have to contend with to a greater extent than was originally thought.

**Disturbances of the earth's natural magnetic field:** for millions of years, every living creature has adapted to tolerate the earth's natural magnetic field. This can be badly distorted by external influences, sometimes evoking spurious controlled responses and even the incorrect regulation of all bodily phenomena.

The main causes of such unnatural field relationships in the bedroom, for example, are metal components in or on the bed – such as internally-sprung mattresses, sprung steel frames and metal bedframes. But steel beams in the structure of the building, radiators, radios, TV sets, quartz alarm clocks, stereo systems and other electrical items in the vicinity of the bed can also have the same effect.

**No metal components in or on the bed**

These magnetic interference fields penetrate most materials, including the tissues of the human body, virtually without hindrance.

**Alternating electric fields:** these are generated when a wire, cable or circuit has a voltage applied to it, even if no lamp or appliance is switched on. In other words, the electrical installation and the appliances connected to it are constantly radiating a certain intrinsic field.

Unfortunately, it usually isn't enough just to take the fuse out of the bedroom's electrical circuit overnight. Other circuits often have an effect on the sleeping area. The only solution to the problem is to install a mains-isolating switch, once a specialist has determined which power circuits have a stressful effect

**Help from a mains-isolating switch**

A mains-isolating switch, which has to be installed by an electrician, costs about £100.

**Alternating magnetic fields:** in addition to electric fields, there are magnetic fields which occur whenever current flows through a cable when an appliance is switched on. They, too, penetrate everything unhindered.

Far too little attention is given to the fact that our health can also be severely stressed by the proximity of high-voltage cables, roof-mounted cable connections and overhead contact wires, and those used on the railways.

**Disturbance of metabolic processes**

### How do rays and energy fields affect our bodies?

There is no doubt that the biochemical and energetic processes in the cells of the body, on which our defence system depends, are adversely affected. Our entire system of glands and hormones, which control innumerable metabolic processes, is sympathetically affected, losing its equilibrium.

The initial consequences of this are vague symptoms that are put down to stress, the weather or other circumstantial factors. If these rays and energy fields continue to affect our bodies after a period of some five to seven years (according to experience), illnesses that are definitely chronic, and often life-threatening, can develop on the same basis: rheumatism, asthma, chronic bronchitis, complaints of the lower abdomen, gastric diseases, gastric ulcers, kidney troubles, nephritis, phlebitis, high blood pressure, irregular heartbeat, myocardial infarction, leukaemia and cancer.

In general, our bodies are weakened by the effects of radiation so that we are no longer properly able to defend ourselves against allergies.

In most cases our homes are over-electrified. The world outside is also affected, not least by the heavy build up of 'weaponry' in the microwave range — TV and radio transmitters, radar systems, radio installations and microwave ovens. All this affects our health and we need to protect ourselves.

### How to have a healthy bedroom

**Simple measures**

To begin with you need to find out whether your sleeping area is affected by the factors already mentioned which could be inflicting consequential, and possibly substantial, harm to your body.

● Obtain the services of a radiesthesist (a dowser) who is also in a position to make a check on electric or electromagnetic fields. The cost will be worthwhile in terms of your health. It is important, however, to be sure to employ someone who is an expert and understands just what the difficulties and problems are in this field.

Be warned against using one of the so-called 'suppressor machines' as some of them are not accurate and will not achieve the desired effect. Ask your dowser whether these pieces of equipment are effective in your home environment.

● Remove all electrical appliances from your sleeping area. At a minimum, pull out the plugs. Invest in a mains-isolating switch and use it during the night. It reduces the voltage across the circuit to four volts (so you can still put the light on). If you have a bedside radio or TV alarm you will need to replace this with a wind-up alarm clock.

● Avoid coiled-spring bed bases, internally sprung mattresses and metal frames. A wooden bed base, with a mattress that contains no metal is better.

● As an allergy sufferer, you need to get rid of everything from your bed and your bedroom to which you may react. This applies above all to animal materials such as feathers, down, wool, sheepskin and horsehair. Latex and futon mattresses are generally compatible, as long as they contain no formaldehyde.

● Absorbent cotton or, if you can afford it silk, make the best bedclothes. Synthetic materials, such as foam-rubber mattresses and synthetic covers, are often recommended for allergy sufferers. However, apart from the fact that they make you more likely to sweat, which is particularly undesirable for eczema patients, many people have an incompatibility to artificial fibres.

**No artificial fibres**

● The same applies to bedding and nightwear. Nightshirts or pyjamas should be labelled: '100% cotton'. 'Pure cotton' can contain a mixture of other textiles.

Make sure that you wash your bed linen with pure soap or soap flakes. The use of caustic detergents and softeners is often a cause of itching at night, especially in cases of eczema. You should also remember that adverse reactions are often provoked by children's cuddly toys.

**Be careful with detergents**

# All ills come from the bowels

It may seem strange in a book about allergies, to have a whole chapter about the bowels, but there is a connection between digestive disorders and the outbreak of an allergy which many people are unaware of. Knowing how the two are connected may help identify certain triggers.

**Irregular digestion**

People commonly think that their digestion is completely normal, but on closer scrutiny all kinds of irregularities come to light. These usually lead to some form of variance from the normal evacuation of a well-shaped, brown stool once a day such as:

- constipation or diarrhoea
- pulpy, unshapely stools
- bright yellow stools
- flatulence
- feelings of repletion
- distended stomach

Pain and colic are less frequent – unfortunately, it must be said, because the result is that people attach little importance to their symptoms because they are not accompanied by acute pain. This means that they neither change their eating habits, nor do they do anything to restore their normal healthy digestion.

**Bowel complaints and other illnesses**

All too often, this opens the door to a large variety of illnesses. These include the true intestinal diseases like gastrointestinal ulcers, inflammation of the colon and gall-bladder complaints, through to cancer of the bowel. But even illnesses such as eczema, migraine, rheumatic complaints and acne are involved here. And we should not forget psychological problems such as depression, mood swings, aggressiveness and lack of motivation .

'The devil is in the bowels,' is a saying common amongst doctors who practise natural medicine. And there is certainly a lot of truth in it. If our bowels are suffering, then there is every liklihood that we are too. To help ourselves we need to understand how our bowels work, what we do that damages them – mostly eating too much and too many of the wrong things – and what we can do to make them, and ourselves better, so that they work more efficiently and we feel healthier.

### How do our digestive organs work?

After we've taken the last bite, we tend not to give any further thought to what happens to the meal that we have just enjoyed. But for our digestive system the hard work has just started. Our bodies have to go through a complicated process in order to extract energy and nutrients from the food we've just eaten.

Strictly speaking, digestion begins in the mouth with the crushing and insalivation of our food. If it is swallowed too quickly and chewed insufficiently – 30 times per bite is the optimum – uncomfortable digestive disorders are quite likely to occur.

**Digestion begins in the mouth**

The stomach, which has a capacity of one and a half litres and is closed off by ring-shaped muscles above and below, is the first stop for food. It stays there for a variable length of time: up to eight hours in the case of sardines in oil, less for easily digested foods. Here, the protein content is predigested by pepsin, an enzyme that is effective only in an acid environment. The hydrochloric acid in the gastric fluid, which fills this role, also kills bacteria.

**Bacteria are killed in the stomach**

The actual work of digestion is done in the small intestine. Three to four metres in length, it lies in many tightly-packed coils, like a tangled ball, in the stomach cavity. To increase the surface area of the mucous membrane it has finger-like projections, the villi, which increase the effective area for digestion from two to 40 square metres – the size of a comfortable flat. The nutrients are piped into the body through the finest blood vessels and a central lymph channel in each villus.

First of all, the nutrients in the chyme (the gruel-like results of gastric digestion) have to be crushed down to their smallest components. To do this, the glands in the mucous membrane of the bowels and the pancreas, secrete digestive juices that split carbohydrates, fats and protein into their smallest particles. The bile, produced by the liver and collected in the gallbladder, makes an important contribution to the digestion of fat. To make the chyme mix more thoroughly, muscle fibres running along the bowel wall make constant small oscillating movements.

Transverse muscle fibres deliver the bowel contents further into the colon by means of wave-like contractions.

The primary task of the colon is to absorb water from the bowel contents so it is not lost to the body. Every day, the body produces three litres of digestive juices alone.

**Bowel bacteria are important to life**

There's something special about the bacteria that populate the colon and the lower part of the small intestine. Their significance was not realized for a long time, then it was discovered that they play an essential role in the digestive process.

They digest the cellulose found in vegetable fibre that hasn't been sufficiently broken down by the digestive juices; they produce vitamins that are vital to us and they train our immune system.

The bacteria, sitting closely-packed together, cover the bowel wall like a carpet.

**Warding off the germs of sickness**

In a reciprocal relationship, they train the lymphatic tissue layer there, thus making a quite essential contribution to warding off the germs of sickness. It's a remarkable fact that 70 per cent of our lymphatic defence system lies in the bowel wall and not, as many people suppose, in the tonsils.

Our digestive apparatus is a very intricate design. It operates automatically, as though under computer control, through our nervous system.

It forgives many a sin at first. But, if we cheat on it repeatedly, the fine interplay of the processes described above loses equilibrium and we have a penalty to pay.

**Sick from careless eating**

We mount the main attacks against the health of our bowels just by wielding a knife and fork. By eating too much and too often, we overload the bowels and overstress the pancreas. In addition, incompletely digested food leads to processes of abnormal gut fermentation and putrefaction. The consequence is increased gas formation, flatulence and feelings of satiation. The gases, which to some extent are absorbed by the body via the bowel wall, stress the liver but primarily they cause headaches, drowsiness, bad moods and depression.

To function optimally, the digestion requires a particular environment, especially in the duodenum which is the topmost part of the small intestine. This environment is determined by the gastric acid. If it is insufficiently acid, the digestive juices from the pancreas can't take full effect and the food is insufficiently digested.

The normal intestinal environment can be further harmed by the chemicals we swallow unknowingly nowadays. These include pesticide residues on our fruit and vegetables, preservatives and antifungal agents and colourants. But it is also harmed by malnourishment caused by the use of white flour instead of wholefood products, by alcohol but, above all, by excess sugar.

**Damage from excess sugar**

The result in the long run is chronic irritation of the intestinal mucus, with consequent inflammatory conditions. The excretory ducts of the gallbladder and the pancreas swell up, further interfering with the operation of the digestive system.

Fostered by these circumstances, allergenic foodstuffs get into the body that would otherwise be trapped by the barrier of the bowels. All the difficulties that occur in the context of a food allergy can develop.

As a result of digestive malfunctions, important minerals such as zinc, manganese, calcium, magnesium and selenium, which, because of intensive farming and over-fertilization of the soil, are already inadequately represented in our food, are absorbed in insufficient quantities. Minerals form components of many enzymes, which are the protein compounds that control the metabolic processes in our bodies. A deficiency will very often show up somewhere other than the bowels.

**Mineral deficiency**

**Vitamin deficiency**

The same applies to vitamins, particularly vitamins B1 and C. The connection between the ensuing symptoms: tiredness, lack of drive, irritation, sleeplessness, calf cramps and depression with their cause – disturbance of the normal conditions in the bowels – is seldom spotted.

And that isn't all; because of the abnormal intestinal environment our intestinal bacteria may be seriously damaged to the detriment of our metabolism.

The intestinal bacteria are also damaged by antibiotics, which, while crusading against all pathogens, can't distinguish between dangerous bacteria and useful ones. This is a good reason for restricting the use of antibiotics to genuinely serious cases of infection.

**Damage to the intestinal flora**

The consequences of damage to the intestinal flora, as the colonies of bacteria in our bowels are termed, are not merely the manifold digestive disorders and deficiency in the vitamins produced by these bacteria, but also loss of the training of our immune system, which raises our susceptibility to infection.

This effect is seen particularly clearly in children who eat too many sweets, which damage their intestinal flora, and as a consequence they are always ill and suffering from colds.

A bowel damaged in this way becomes infested with bacteria that harm rather than help us. Moreover, fungi, particularly the thrush fungus (candida albicans), spread at an increasing rate.

**Fungal infection**

Most people then suffer from smeary stools with occasional mucus layers, strong flatulence, diarrhoea or constipation and occasional cramp-like stomach pains. Since the fungi are a drain on the vitamins in food, the existing vitamin deficiency is further intensified.

By fermenting sugar and other carbohydrates, fungi also cause various fusel alcohols to appear. These make patients feel slightly befuddled all the time. If they then drink a glass of wine, they become tipsy faster than usual and are surprised to find how little they can take.

### How to sort out your bowels

Unfortunately, the easiest method, and the one most people are accustomed to – taking a pill three times a day – does not work.

**Patience and persistence**

If you genuinely want to make your bowels healthy again your require two things: patience and persistence. What you've vandalized through years of abuse can't be rebuilt in the twinkling of an eye. So expect to spend months at least, under the guidance of a doctor with experience in intestinal rehabilitation, aiming at a goal which, in the interest of your health, is truly worthwhile. Once that goal is achieved you will feel much better and your bowels will be healthier, creating a positive impact on your allergy.

### Bowel treatment - step by step

**A change of diet:** is an indispensable prerequisite. Above all, you must avoid sugar, white flour products, alcohol and pork (including sausages). Eat as few sweet things as possible. If absolutely necessary, use sweeteners (from health-food shops or a chemist), honey, pear syrup, maple syrup or dried sugar-cane juice as alternatives.

**Wholefood diet**

Change your diet to wholefoods and include a considerable proportion of raw foods in your diet each day so that the intestinal bacteria are nourished and will flourish again. But, while doing this, you should exclude your food allergens and do without anything that's stodgy or causes you discomfort.

It is best to avoid the radical and abrupt dietary changes that some regimes propose. Flatulence, feelings of satiation or stomach pains are a sign that your damaged bowels can't cope with the raw food which, though healthy, is unfamiliar.

In this event, eat whole grains for the first four weeks, cooked as a grain soup, before you change over to muesli as your morning dish. You may also have to begin with cooked vegetables before you're able to switch to raw salads. Start with a few trial bites before a cooked meal, and gradually build up the amount. Chew thoroughly, eat little, and don't overload your stomach and bowels. Give them four hours rest between meals.

**Chew thoroughly**

**A stool examination:** you can ask your doctor to have this done in a specialist laboratory. The analysis gives information about your intestinal flora. The findings will tell your doctor how things are going with your intestinal bacteria, what healthy ones have survived, whether there is an overgrowth of pathogenic ones and, above all, whether fungi or protozoa (lamblia intestinalis or amoebas) have been detected. These latter particularly enjoy colonizing a damaged bowel.

If found, any fungi and protozoa must first be eliminated **Rebuilding** by the appropriate means prescribed by your doctor. Special **healthy** bacterial preparations will then ensure that a normal **intestinal** intestinal flora will be rebuilt. The process has to be gone **flora** through slowly and gradually.

Partial components or the metabolic products of bacteria are added first, and later the appropriate bacterial cultures. The preparations available are used in accordance with the doctor's experience and judgement. They include a variety of preparations that can reseed the gut with normal bowel bacteria to re-establish a healthy fermentation process. These products are called probiotics. Acidophillus preparations are the most commonly available probiotics.

For relief you can take Sanoghurt, Bioghurt or Biogarde and lactose (1-2 teaspoons of lactose per pot), but only **Be careful** provided you have no incompatibility with dairy products or **with dairy** lactose. Lactose intolerance can be tested as described in **products** testing for food allergies (page 66).

# Allergic illnesses

## Hay fever

It's usually in the warmest months of the year, the months people look forward to all through a cold winter, that hay fever strikes its victims.

As a rule, hay fever develops at pre-school or school age. Very young children and babies don't usually develop it, but once you have it you will probably go on suffering until you are over 50 years of age. This is a very good reason to declare war on this affliction at an early stage.

### How does hay fever come about?

Although, from its name, it sounds as though it is hay that causes hay fever, it isn't just hay that turns the spring and summer into torture for hypersensitive people. Hay fever is **Pollen –** mainly caused by the pollens of grass, weeds, shrubs, trees **February to** and – more rarely – flowers. For many, the suffering begins **September** in February and often doesn't end until September.

### What are the symptoms?

Symptoms include a tickling sensation in the nose; itchiness, tickling or a sore feeling in the throat; explosive sneezes, but above all a running nose that slowly but surely turns bright red. Nasal secretions are watery and clear. If they turn yellow, this usually indicates a festering infection, which in turn could mean a chronic infection of the nasal passages.

The eyes, too, are usually red, itchy and sometimes weeping. Sometimes the ears or the mucous membranes of the genitals also feel itchy. In children, an uncontrollable attack of coughing sometimes follows an allergic **The effect on** inflammation of the tonsils which may be mistaken for **children** whooping cough.

General well-being is almost always adversely affected. You will feel tired, irritated, nervous, drained of energy, shivery, and may sleep badly because your nose is swollen and blocked. Swallowed pollen can also affect the intestinal mucous membrane, causing diarrhoea and stomach pains.

True hay fever is associated with spring and summer

**Combined with other allergies**

and, in some cases, autumn, too. If it persists after that time, then a combination with some other allergen, such as fungi and mites, is more than likely. A doctor should make a diagnosis although the symptoms usually speak for themselves. The prick test (page 16) is a good indicator of the range of pollens that may be the cause.

**Leave diagnosis to the doctor**

### Conventional therapy

There are over-the-counter remedies which are available from a chemist, but also seek advice from your doctor.

**In acute conditions:** brief respite can be had by means of antihistamines, as tablets or drops. They switch the allergic reaction off. Newer preparations have the advantage of not causing drowsiness.

Hyposensitization is a long-term treatment which used to be very popular, but is now not commonly used. The individual allergens are identified and the body is desensitized by injecting them subcutaneously in small quantities of increasing concentration.

**Desensitize the body**

This treatment usually takes three years. Your doctor will begin with the injections in late autumn, especially if you are allergic to early-flowering plants. The success achieved varies: it depends on the precision with which the range of allergens is detected by the tests. The wider your range of allergens, the greater the risk that some allergens will not have been detected. These are likely to be responsible for the continued existence of your hay fever. They may be other grass or flower pollens, but are likely to be different allergens such as fungi, house dust, mites or animal hairs.

Successful treatment does not mean that you will now be immune to the formation of a reaction to new allergens. It is quite likely that other allergens will affect you.

### Natural therapy

**Homeopathy:** *luffa operculata* is a South American gourd plant which forms the basis for most hay-fever remedies.

*Galphimia glauca*, a Mexican medicinal plant, is well known for treating allergic reactions of the skin and mucous

**Natural remedies**

membranes, and is also used for hay fever. This remedy can be taken in C6 potency, three to five times a day as a preventative measure. There are also a large number of homeopathic mixtures available for the treatment of hay fever and these should be taken as indicated. They can be obtained in most health food shops and many pharmacies.

**Vegetable agents:** *eccinacea* can be taken in the acute stage. Take it as two capsules initially, reducing to one, three times a day in each case.

**Acupuncture:** this method has proved very useful as a back-up to other measures. Some of the points of application are on the face, close to the wings of the nostrils. Since this area is very sensitive, it is worth having the acupuncture done with a laser beam rather than needles (page 76).

**The painless laser beam**

**Formic acid:** *acidum formicium* also has a beneficial effect in the case of allergic illnesses. An appropriate preparation (C6, or even C30) can be given orally.

The homeopathic constitutional agent (page 73), which must be individually formulated by an experienced homeopath, can improve hay fever. As back-up, a homeopathic pollen preparation, such as pollen C6 or C30 can be taken as a preventive from as early as January onward. If hay fever has already broken out, increase the dose of five drops from three times daily to five times a day.

You can try some non-homeopathic pollen preparations, such as propolis. This should be taken over a prolonged period of time, starting in winter. It works by gradually making the body insensitive by accustoming it to the pollen.

A similar result can be obtained by regularly taking doses of high-quality honey, which comes if possible from near where you live, so that it contains the same pollens as the ones that affect you. Three months before the anticipated outbreak of hay fever, take a tablespoon of honey (comb honey is best) after every meal and, before going to bed, take a further tablespoon of it in half a glass of warm water.

**Pollen preparations**

Then, two weeks before your hay fever season starts, take two teaspoons of honey and two teaspoons of fruit vinegar in half a glass or, if you prefer, a full glass of water, before breakfast and before going to bed at night.

**Pollen preparations**

**Honey and fruit vinegar**

This treatment should be taken every day throughout the hay-fever period. You should also keep on taking the tablespoon of honey after your lunch and again after your evening meal.

Chewing pieces of honeycomb as many times a day as necessary will also help keep your nose clear. You should take a piece of honeycomb, the size of a piece of chewing gum, and chew it for around 15 minutes, at hourly intervals.

Chewing honeycomb is also thought to have a healing effect in cases of chronic sinusitis and inflammation in the mouth.

**Honeycomb**

There are things you can do to help yourself before going to your doctor for treatment: try homeopathic treatment using the hay-fever remedies. Take doses of Eccinacea, honey and fruit vinegar. Avoid milk and dairy products as you may have a latent allergy to milk which will aggravate your hay fever.

### General rules for living

**Avoid the allergens:** you won't be able to avoid pollen completely unless you move to the Arctic or more than 5,000m up a mountain. All the same, how badly you suffer will depend on how much pollen there is around to attack your mucous membranes. You'll find a few tips to protect yourself, to some extent at least, in the following section on asthma.

**Avoid milk:** try to avoid milk, at least during the hay fever season. Hay fever sufferers often have a latent milk allergy that has escaped detection so, if the body is relieved of this factor, it is then better able to deal with pollens.

Initially you should avoid all dairy products and also ensure that you don't take them in as unnoticed additives. If your symptoms improve, you can see whether they get

Milk allergy
is the
foundation

worse again when you introduce a moderate amount of milk products back into your diet. If they do, try goats' or sheep's milk, or go without milk entirely during the relevant months.

If you want to do your body more good, set aside a few days every so often when you only eat raw fruit and vegetables, and, in between times, ensure that salads and fruit make up at least one quarter of your daily menu.

## Asthma

This tormenting illness requires the intensive use of natural healing methods, which are most effective when used together.

Take
immediate
action

Once the illness has taken hold, it is very difficult to cure. Only well-targeted therapy, applied when the first symptoms appear, can be really effective.

### How does asthma come about?

This allergy often has a basis in hereditary over-sensitivity. As a rule, patients react to a variety of materials such as pollen, fungi, mites, house dust, contact with animals or cigarette smoke. Latent food allergies, such as milk allergy, are involved more often than is generally supposed (page 66).

On the other hand there are also cases in which infectious diseases caused by viruses or bacteria prepare the way for asthma (infectious asthma). Although mental conflicts, or stress, can have an adverse effect and an attack can even be triggered by a confrontation with your boss or trouble with your mother-in-law, asthma is primarily not a psychogenic illness. In other words, stress makes things worse, but isn't the basic cause.

Bacteria and
viruses

Similarly, where asthma exists, an attack can be triggered by physical exertion (exercise-induced asthma).

### How does asthma reveal itself?

Coughing, expectoration and shortness of breath result from a constriction of the bronchi (as a consequence of spasm of the fine muscle fibres in the bronchial walls) and mucous congestion.

It's mainly exhalation of air from the pulmonary alveoli that is hampered, whereas, in croup, which often afflicts young children, a wheezing noise is heard during inhalation and the lips can take on a bluish tinge for lack of oxygen.

In chronic asthma the ribcage may become deformed and take on a barrel-shaped appearance with the ribs standing out horizontally.

### Conventional therapy

In this illness, too, conventional therapy is limited to the relief of the symptoms without being able to contribute to genuine healing. But conventional medicines can give considerable relief from the tormenting shortness of breath which is suffered during a serious asthma attack.

One of the main types of medication used in conventional therapy, which can only be carried out by a doctor, are reliever inhalers which contain drugs like terbutaline or salbutamol. These should always be kept at hand so that they can be taken at the first sign of any symptoms developing.

**Relief of symptoms**

If a reliever inhaler has to be used more than once a day, then you may be given an inhaled 'preventer' medicine such as a corticosteriod.

If your asthma needs further control another bronchodilator, which relaxes and opens the narrowed airways, such as salmeterol may be given as well.

If the symptoms still need controlling beta$_2$-adrenoceptor stimulants may be given by mouth. These open up the airways, make the heart beat faster and the blood vessels dilate so that the blood flows more easily around the body.

**Relievers and preventers**

In severe asthma a course of corticosteroid tablets may be necessary from time to time, but would only be considered for long-term treatment if other treatments proved inadequate.

The primary aim of treatment is to free the patient from discomfort using the remedies stated, avoiding steroids wherever possible, so that unrestrained asthma does not develop. This happens when the bronchi alter over a period of time and the vegetative nervous system is not correctly controlled. This condition becomes more serious, even irreversible, the longer asthma continues.

Natural therapy should initially accompany conventional medication. If there is an improvement, you can gradually try to do without the medicines.

### Natural Therapy
In an acute case it is often necessary to start off with some form of conventional remedy to allay the symptoms.

Natural and orthodox medicines

Any homeopathic remedies should be individually selected by a homeopath, so only a rough overview can be given here:

*Arsenicum C30* provides relief if a serious attack of asthma, occurring between midnight and three in the morning, is combined with fear and agitation and the patient is suffering from shortness of breath which is accompanied by severe bouts of coughing.

*Ipecacuanha* (especially useful for treating children) should be used where there is mucous congestion on the chest which is accompanied by heavy, rattling breathing.

*Tartarus emeticus* can be taken for slight wheezing, pallor and impending pneumonia.

*Coccus cacti* for convulsive coughing with abundant stringy, tough mucus.

*Natrium sulfuricum* for asthma which occurs in a damp environment and is aggravated by rain or mist.

*Teucrium* should be taken if the condition appears to worsen in the autumn.

*Ambra or Ignatia* where asthma occurs as a result of grief, worries or injury.

In some cases complex preparations, prepared from ready-made mixtures of two or more homeopathic remedies, may be recommended.

As with illnesses other than asthma, only the

homeopathic constitutional agent (page 74) has a profound effect. It must be individually devised by an experienced homeopath.

Treatment by a homeopath

The following herb teas are recommended for asthma and convulsive bronchitis: a mixture of coltsfoot leaves, ribwort, fennel, thyme and melissa in equal parts. A herbalist will prepare the mixture for you. Pour ¼ litre of boiling water over two teaspoons of the mixture, allow it to stand for ten minutes, strain and sweeten with honey. Drink one cup three to five times a day.

**Simple remedies**

A lemon compress will help relieve bronchial spasms. First soak a cotton or linen cloth with pure lemon juice, and then lay it on a towel which is large enough to enclose and cover the upper part of the body. Fold the compress over the chest. It can be left on for several hours.

A quark compress has the same effect. Use a nappy or something similar for the innermost layer and spread half of it with low-fat quark, at room temperature, to a thickness of 1 cm. Then fold the other half over it. Cover this with a piece of towelling and some thin, woollen material. The compress can be left on for an hour or, if applied in the evening, it can be left in place overnight.

### Nutritional medicine

Asthma sufferers frequently have low levels of essential nutrients. The addition of magnesium (400-800mg per day), vitamin C (1000-2000 mg per day), selenium (200 mcg per day) zinc, (50mg per day), vitamin B (50mg per day) and vitamin B6 (50mg per day) can be of great benefit to asthma sufferers.

Ideally any vitamin and mineral therapy should be discussed in detail with a trained nutitional therapist or doctor before you start.

**Under medical supervision**

### Breathing exercises

While asthma is not primarily a physcological illness, stress can play an important role. Breathing exercises based on relaxation techniques, such as those used in yoga, can be of great benefit to asthma sufferers.

### Desensitization

Many asthmatics with inhaled, contact or chemical sensitivities cannot completely avoid contact with their allergens – such as pollen or mould. There are three major methods of desensitization available within complementary medicine: Isopathic, Miller technique desensitization and Enzyme potentiated desnsitization.

Isopathic desensitization involves the patient taking a homeopathic potency of the substance to which they are allergic. If they suffer from hay fever due to birch pollen, then this means taking a dilution of birch pollen in homoepathic potency. The exact dilution will need to be prescribed by a competent homeopath or allergist, and will often need to be taken either continuously or intermittently for a period of between three to 12 months. There is some interesting and provocative evidence of the effectiveness of isopathic desensitization, making it one of the few areas of homeopathy that has hard evidence to support it.

Miller technique desensitization involves allergens being diluted wiith salt water on a 1:5 basis thereby making up a set of serially diluted containers, each with progressively less allergen than the last. These dilutions can then either be injected into the patient's skin or given to the patient sublingually in order to test for an allergic response. As the patient takes a chemical food or other allergen in decreasing dilutions, he will note that if the substance is injected a positive skin reaction will occur, often associated with the symptoms triggered by that particular allergen. This usually occurs in the lower dilutions and not immediately with the high concentrates of allergen. In other words, the Miller technique has something in common with homeopathy, but is not a true homeopathic medicine. Once the dilution that provoked a positive skin reaction or appropriate symptoms has been identified, then regularly taking a dose slightly below that (the underdose) can cause an overall improvement in symptoms.

The aim of Miller technique desensitization is therefore to provoke symptoms with a particular allergen in order to clarify the diagnosis and then to use it therapeutically by

**Three major methods**

giving the neutralizing does of allergen. This techniqe is widely utilized by those practising environmental medicine, and requires the patient to take desensitizing medication for a period of between six and 18 months in order to overcome their allergies. The dilutions used therapeutically may need to be checked and changed from time to time by the doctor providing the treatment, but this technique has very broad applications and can be utilized in conditions where it is impossible to completely avoid the allergen which may be provoking your symptoms.

**Provoke symptoms**

Enzyme potentiated desensitization was developed by Dr Len McEwen, who originally conceived of the idea while he was a pharmacologist at St Mary's Hospital Medical School, London. The method consists of injecting very highly purified antigens in miniscule doses, along with an enzyme called beta-glucuronidase which increases the effects of the injected antigens. The technique appears to change patients' immune thermostat over quite a prolonged period of time; they gradually become less food and environment sensitive, but this may take a period of between one and three years. The technique is safe, and there have been some encouraging clinical trails of the use of this technique in a variety of conditions such as arthritis, eczema and colitis.

The technique itself can only be provided by an appropriately qualified registered medical practitioner. An initial course of EDP will usually involve between three and five injections, given once every two months, and you will then be able to assess whether the treatment is proving effective for you after a six to ten month period. You may need to go on having injections once every six to twelve months.

**Qualified practitioner**

Acupuncture should be used whenever possible if chronic asthma needs to be brought under control.

**Laser treatment is painless**

It requires 15 to 20 weekly sessions. For children, a laser, which is a painless, can be used instead of needles. Acupuncture is worth looking at as a treatment for children because they normally respond particularly well to this type of regulatory therapy.

Acupuncture should, of course, be combined with other appropriate measures so that the illness is attacked from several directions. In this way a greater effect is far more likely to be obtained.

Mental stability is particularly important in asthma sufferers, since negative emotions can have an adverse effect on the illness. It is important to keep your lifestyle as free as possible from stress and conflict. This applies to both your home and working environment. Things that you can do to help contribute to your own mental harmonization are mentioned elsewhere (page 96)

**Ensure mental harmony**

In addition, hypnosis has time and again proven itself effective against asthma. It should be carried out by a trained specialist, usually a psychologist, psychiatrist or hypnotherapist.

It is a pity that this highly effective method of treatment is often viewed with suspicion because of its misuse as a form of entertainment and all the attendant publicity it receives In the hands of a knowledgeableand responsible person, hypnosis is a completely safe method of affecting our subconscious and the vegetative nervous system that the latter controls. Both play a major role in the course of the disease.

These are some self-help remedies to try before medical therapy:
Drink herb tea made of coltsfoot, ribwort, fennel, thyme or melissa.
Apply a lemon or quark compress.
Do breathing exercises (after obtaining guidance from a physiotherapist).
Take a homeopathic remedy.

## General Rules for Living
**Avoid allergens:** this isn't easy for asthma sufferers, but every effort you can make to avoid allergens is worthwhile, as it will save your body from a confrontation.

Besides pollen in the case of pollen asthma, particular attention should be given to fungi, mites, house dust, animal hairs and skin particles, besides job-related causes such as mill dust in the case of millers' asthma.

**Check your food** **Nutrition:** remember that a food sensitivity is a common trigger (page 67) and the relevant food should be eliminated from your diet, either temporarily or permanently. Any foods that contain invisible fungi, or are produced using fungal enzymes should be regarded with suspicion (page 19).

**Medication:** a number of medicines contain substances that can trigger asthma, such as sulphites in remedies for vomiting, in antibiotics, psychopharmaceuticals, painkillers and bronchi expanding medicines. If you have to keep taking these medicines, check with the manufacturers. Even aspirin in painkillers or flu medicines and morphine may be incompatible with your system. **Be careful with medicines**

**Humidifiers:** these often blow fungi or bacteria into the air. Inhalers, too, need to be cleaned regularly and carefully.

**Tobacco smoke:** this is pure poison for an asthma sufferer. Although in the strict sense the smoke is not an allergen, every irritation by chemical substances in the inhaled air (and this applies largely to tobacco smoke, which even contains formaldehyde) can set up, or trigger, the next asthmatic attack.

**Tobacco smoke is pure poison** The harmful effects of smoking damage both active and passive smokers. It isn't just people who have asthma who suffer either. Nervousness, irritation and disturbed concentration are just some of the unwelcome effects that smokers impose on others around them.

Although there is no doubt that it is difficult to stop smoking, there are a number of ways that you can help yourself (acupuncture is just one of them). The effect that smoking has on others really amounts to physical injury.

In principle there should be no smoking in the home of an asthmatic person, because they could be sensitive to even the smallest amount of smoke, which stays suspended in the air even after a room has been ventilated.

This applies even if no direct effects of smoke can be observed in the patient.

**Infections:** these worsen the suffering of many an asthmatic person. Chronic sinusitis, which is common in asthma patients, also plays a role here and it should be treated with natural methods, not antibiotics. Acupuncture, herbal or homeopathic agents can all be used as a cure. It is very important that asthma sufferers avoid catching colds.

The following may also be helpful: a weekly trip to the sauna; hydrotherapy treatment; brush massage, taking a preparation containing Eccinacea, or taiga root from Russia.

## Eczema

This agonizing illness is becoming increasingly common in a very worrying way. Even very young babies and small children can be affected, with the effects being seen all over their bodies.

The inability of conventional medicine to provide a genuine cure is especially regrettable in view of the psychological strain suffered by affected people, who have **Other** external disfigurement and an excruciating itch. This is what **remedies** makes patients set off on a real odyssey from doctor to doctor, from non-medical practitioner to faith healer, trying everything that promises help. Self-help groups have been formed by suffers in an effort to find help and support.

More than anything else, eczema clearly illustrates the fact that a sickness usually has deeper roots than are suggested by its outward appearance. Contributing factors can include malfunction of the pancreas, spleen and liver, a damaged bowel, weakened defensive powers and mineral deficiency, among others.

Here, again, it becomes evident that natural holistic **A sickness** treatment, since it attacks from more than one direction, is **with deeper** superior to purely local treatment. From the natural healing **roots** point of view, eczema is a systemic illness rather than a skin disease, and should therefore be treated holistically.

### How does eczema come about?

Usually a genetic predisposition is to blame. It may show itself in other members of the family in the form of other allergic illnesses such as hay fever, asthma or in some cases as a food allergy.

**Genetic factor**

Clues indicating a genetic factor include dry skin and a double transverse fold below the eyelids. Even newborn babies can show an increase in typical immunoglobulins in the blood of the umbilical cord. Whether this leads to the actual illness depends largely on the extent to which the body is assaulted by other factors such as malnourishment, environmental contamination or contact with animals.

### How does eczema reveal itself?

The most prominent feature is reddening of the skin, which is usually somewhat swollen with a tendency to flakiness. Sometimes there is a persistent discharge from particular spots, or colonization of the injured areas of skin by pus bacteria, herpes viruses or fungi.

**Cradle cap**

In small children, the cheeks are often affected or sometimes there is cradle cap. Later, apart from the face, it is mainly the throat, neck, the bend of the elbows, the hollows of the knees, wrists and ankles that are affected. The skin lesions, however, can also spread to the trunk and all along the arms and legs.

**Tormenting itch**

The endless torment comes mainly from the accompanying itch. This can often stop the person getting to sleep and, after nights of sleep deprivation, finally turns him or her into a real bundle of nerves.

### Conventional therapy

As a rule, this is applied externally in the form of treatment with ointment, with or without cortisone. Cortisone ointments, however, are being refused by an increasing number of patients who have noticed that, when treatment ends, the skin damage and itch often return worse than they were before.

**Beware of asthma**

Alarm is justified if, when the skin rash has been suppressed, asthma puts in an appearance.

**Natural therapy**

Diet is the central pillar of any treatment intended to lead to lasting improvement or freedom from symptoms. Contrary to traditional opinion, eczema is almost invariably based on food incompatibility.

It is usually latent, however, only becoming clearly recognizable when a trial fast is carried out or an elimination diet, consisting of only a few foods that are above suspicion, is followed (page 64). For this to work the skin must not be treated with ointment. Any improvement can then be confidently ascribed to the diet. Even homeopathic agents should not be taken during this period. In most patients the skin heals up and the itch is eased when the elimination diet is completed. The effect is especially rapid in children.

**Elimination diet**

Gradually, one food after another should be reintroduced into the menu and the patient observed for any resulting deterioration. If there is any, the food concerned is erased from the diet. There's more detailed information in the chapter on Food Allergy (page 62).

It's important to wait until the improvement in the skin has progressed far enough to make any deterioration unmistakable. It isn't necessary to wait for complete healing, which would take too long, but a clearly observable reduction should have set in.

The original bright redness changes to a more bluish red, the swelling also lessens and the skin begins to flake heavily. This is a clear sign of improvement, because it's the diseased surface layers of skin that are flaking off. Tender new skin, free of inflammation, appears underneath. When you run your hand over it, it feels soft. Moreover, it's particularly well supplied with circulating blood. Typically, the colour of the skin changes dramatically: in conditions of heat, sweat, emotion or physical activity it can redden noticeably and, on cooling or when excited, it can go pale. By contrast, the redness of inflammation remains constant. Simply because the skin has a better supply of blood, the accompanying itch is cured. Before starting to test the next food, it's imperative that you await further improvement -

**Flaking skin is a good sign**

**Careful trial**

not only at the beginning but also, if deterioration has appeared, after testing a food. The results of the elimination diet are so good that a careful trial always pays off.

The connection with an individual's own food incompatibility can be impressively and convincingly shown in this way because the skin serves as an obvious witness here. This is particularly true in children. Adults, on the other hand, are often subject to additional causative factors that need to be taken into consideration.

Patients with serious eczema are well advised to adapt to the elimination diet in a specialist clinic, especially after treatment with cortisone.

**Lack of minerals**

People who have eczema – like those who have a food allergy – are often deficient in a number of vital substances, such as minerals and trace elements, and sometimes also in vitamins. This is especially so in the cases of calcium, magnesium, zinc, selenium, manganese and vitamins B and C. It is therefore a good idea to supply any minerals and trace elements or vitamins that are lacking, at least for a while at the start of a treatment, under the supervision of your doctor.

**Microbiological bowel therapy:** as has already been explained, the normal intestinal bacteria are often disturbed in allergy sufferers. It is consequently possible to observe that the skin, for example, often deteriorates following a bout of intestinal flu. Success in treating eczema, therefore, can often be achieved simply by administering a preparation that rebuilds the intestinal flora (page 39).

**Acupuncture:** this ancient Chinese treatment often has a beneficial effect, but primarily when used as a supportive therapy ( page 75).

**Homeopathic remedies:** improvement can often be achieved with these, especially with some homeopathic constitutional agents.

**Extensive experience is required**

A homeopath dealing with cases of eczema needs to have extensive experience, because deterioration in the form of excessive initial reactions can very easily occur, for example when high potencies of sulphur are used (page 73).

**Local treatment:** local treatment of skin lesions must take second place to general treatment. Eczema has to heal from within, not by suppression of the symptoms from outside. This especially applies to serious cases. In less serious cases, if the patient feels his skin to be tense and unpleasantly dry, ointment (in the smallest possible amount) may be used for treatment. Compatibility varies between different kinds of ointment.

There are three main reasons why using as little ointment as possible is advisable:

● The pores become blocked and skin respiration suffers.

● Each preparation entails a risk of incompatibility, especially if it contains vegetable substances, particularly camomile or marigold.

● If a food-allergy test is being made, skin reactions can no longer be interpreted with confidence – improvement or deterioration might be due to the ointment.

**Use as little ointment as possible**

**Try simple moisturizing creams**

Try and use simple moisturizing creams such as E45. Calendula cream can also help healing and may alleviate the itching. Try as far as possible to avoid creams containing cortisone or steroids.

Sometimes quite a simple and cheap measure — just dabbing the skin with a good, cold-pressed olive oil — is enough to give relief. You can also put some in your washing or into your bath water.

Adding salt from the Dead Sea to your bath also soothes the itch: you can get it from the chemist. It dries the skin out slightly, however, with an initial burning sensation where there are open spots.

You can make compresses with pansy tea instead: pour 2 litre of boiling water over two teaspoons of the stems and leaves, but don't strain the resulting mixture. Soak a linen cloth with the brew. Lay the cloth on the affected area and cover it with a dry cloth. Repeat the compress frequently.

**Compresses**

Try some of these before seeking medical treatment:
● Make a bath or a compress with a pansy brew or with salt from the Dead Sea.
● Rub in calendula cream to counter the itch.
● Give the elimination diet a try.

### General rules for living

The sufferer from eczema should do some detective work to track down and eradicate all the things that could irritate his skin – and there are a lot of these.

Here are the most important points that you need to bear in mind:

**Do not wear wool**

**Clothing:** wool should be avoided by patients and by other family members who have contact with them. A mother who takes her child who is suffering from eczema in her arms, for example, should not wear a woolly pullover.

Many sufferers also find synthetic fibres unbearable. Textiles often contain a small, and sometimes undeclared, amount of these fibres. Seams sewn with artificial fibres can be recognized by their bright appearance, even when lighting conditions are poor.

The most compatible materials are silk and cotton. The latter, however, is often treated with formaldehyde (starch and anti-creasing agents). You should wash new cotton things four times: a single wash often brings out the formaldehyde content even more strongly.

Reactions can also be provoked by cleaning solvents, a small amount of which always remains in the clothing. Select clothing that you can wash, rather than items that require dry cleaning. Textile dyes, too, can sometimes provoke allergies.

It's important to wear underclothes and stockings that absorb sweat well. Here, too, cotton has proved its worth.

Shoe leather and sports shoes are often chemically treated. Take note of this if you have reddened areas of skin on your feet. Rubber boots, too, can cause skin symptoms.

If your feet are affected, wear sandals or very low-cut shoes and, at home, pad around in thick cotton socks or bare feet.

**Bedclothes:** more details have already been given in the chapter on 'What triggers allergies? (see page 18). Don't use any materials containing sheep's wool or horsehair. You also need to be careful with foam-rubber mattresses and synthetic-fibre covers, which cause more sweating in eczema sufferers. The best thing is a mattress made from vegetable material (kapok) and a cotton or silk bedspread. The housedust mite is a particularly important trigger for eczema.

**Detergents:** common detergents, including biological and phosphate-free ones, often cause skin reactions in eczema sufferers. It is best, therefore, to do your washing with neutral soap or soap flakes. Don't use softeners but, instead, put a little vinegar into the rinsing water. If you use a tumble drier, your washing will still stay soft. Bed linen, too, should be washed in the same way. For highly sensitive people, washing should be rinsed several times. Make your washing machine go through the rinse cycle at least one more time.

**Personal hygiene:** make it a rule not to use products containing preservatives or herbal additives. Herbs such as camomile and St John's wort are often incompatible.

Use hypoallergenic products, particularly when considering soap and other cleansing creams. Face creams which contain fats and moisture also have good compatibility. Every brand of toothpaste contains a number of additives that could provoke an allergic reaction. Careful brushing with pure water for at least three minutes is enough, plus perhaps a weekly cleaning with calcium carbonate (obtainable from the chemist).

*Be aware of skin symptoms*

**Tap water:** unfortunately, even tap water is incompatible in many respects because of the impurities and additives it contains. It causes reddening of the skin and itching in eczema sufferers whenever they shower or wash.

**Don't wash too frequently**

This is not an excuse not to avoid washing of course, but you should reduce your contact with water to the minimum., so don't take a bath or shower every day. Desensitization may help with tap water sensitivity.

Bath oils may contain groundnut or soya oil, which many allergy sufferers can't tolerate. Babies and small children can be washed with bottled spring water if money is not a problem and you don't have to count the pennies.

**Avoid cosmetics and perfume**

As far as possible avoid all cosmetics and perfumes. The less your body comes into contact with chemical products, the better off you will be.

If, however, you're unwilling to do without your favourite fragrance or a pleasantly aromatic body lotion after your bath or shower, then do test the products very carefully. Eliminate all cosmetics for a while, then reintroduce your favourites one at a time, on trial. The important thing here is to make sure you allow gaps of several days between each one in order to see whether an incompatibility reaction occurs.

Remember, too, that you can become allergic to a product with which you previously had no difficulty.

**Animals:** as a rule, a household containing an allergic person should keep no pets (page 23). Allergy sufferers should stay away from places where animals and birds are kept, such as a zoo.

**Domestic poisons:** formaldehyde from furniture, chipboard, glued carpets and the wood preservatives used in windows, timber cladding and ceilings, always forms a basis for the occurrence of eczema.

Just as in the case of asthma or chronic susceptibility to infection, you should consider these possible causes if, even after applying natural treatment, you haven't achieved a breakthrough cure.

**In the case of children:** you have to bear some more things in mind. Playing in the sand or contact with snow, soft toys, plastic toys or handicraft materials such as adhesives or modelling clay can provoke allergic skin reactions. Plastic pacifiers (dummies) can cause extensive facial eczema.

Careful observation is required

## Food allergy

### An illness with many faces

The symptoms of a food allergy differ so much from person to person and range so widely and variously, literally from head to toe, that the person affected usually never realizes they could be associated with his diet.

*Symptoms from top to toe*

Normally you would suppose that foods that are incompatible must manifest themselves by the disturbances they cause in the digestive organs. Although this happens, these digestive disturbances are so minor that often no attention is paid to them.

On the other hand there are many symptoms which you normally wouldn't associate with eating, either because they're so general and unspecific, like tiredness or nervousness, or because their connection with the bowels is far from obvious, as with joint pains, headaches and a racing heartbeat.

*Unspecific symptoms*

There is also the additional difficulty that no time connection can be discerned between the intake of a particular food and the occurrence of symptoms even when that food is eaten daily.

Often, food incompatibility is not the only cause, though it is usually the fundamental, reason for complaints and illnesses.

*Is food allergy the cause?*

These include:
- excess weight
- migraine
- gastrointestinal illnesses
- high/low blood pressure
- asthma
- rheumatic joint pains
- Eczema
- psoriasis
- susceptibility to infection
- hyperactivity in children
- depression
- addictive illnesses.

**There are usually several symptoms**

The fact that these illnesses can have a common root, namely a food allergy, is shown not only by the success obtained with a low-allergen diet, but also by the observation that they can occur in combination in one and the same person. Alternatively, in one family, the mother may suffer from migraine, the child from eczema, asthma or hyperactivity and the aunt from depression, while the uncle is overweight.

It is unclear why food allergy should manifest itself in such different ways. Perhaps it has to do with the fact that each of us is an individual and our organisms have their own separate set of weak points

A food allergy rarely confines itself to one symptom. Usually we see several of the complaints described below which are also subject to change. So check the list carefully. Not every sufferer has all the symptoms mentioned, of course. But, if you observe three or more of them in yourself, there are grounds for suspecting that you have a food allergy, and it's worth giving the dietary test a try.

Each of the symptoms listed below can have completely different causes, of course, and these must be clarified in every case by relevant investigation. But a patient's poor state of health is often in total contrast with clear laboratory findings. This can often lead a doctor to regard the symptoms as psychological, rather than physical in origin.

**Ill, no matter what the laboratory results say**

**General complaints:** chronic fatigue, lassitude, lack of energy, listlessness, cold feelings from within, shivers down the spine, pallor, tingling in the hands, occasional facial swellings (oedemas) on the eyelids, hands and ankles, for example, sweating even in the absence of exertion, headaches, dizziness, excess weight or weight deficiency, wide fluctuations in weight over one's lifetime, and raised temperature.

**The mind is affected, too**

**Mental disturbances:** aggression, nervousness, inner agitation, hyperactivity, lack of concentration, poor memory, drowsiness, inability to think clearly, confusion, apathy, lack of drive, speech disorders, irritability, states of anxiety and panic, depression, impaired appetite often accompanied by obsessional eating.

**Sense organs:** blocked or watery running nose, chronic sinusitis, bouts of sneezing, conjunctivitis, dark circles round the eyes, blurred vision, tinnitus and frequent ear inflammation.

**Skin:** itch, eczema (neurodermatitis), nettle rash (urticaria), psoriasis and other skin rashes.

**Head:** chronic headaches, migraine.

**Digestive organs:** aphthous ulcers in the mouth, gastric and duodenal ulcers, flatulence, stomach pains, chronic constipation or diarrhoea, anal eczema, chronic diseases of the colon.

**Possible physical complaints**

**Heart and circulation:** low or high blood pressure, pressure or pains in the left half of the chest, slow or (especially) fast pulse, racing heartbeat and fainting fits.

**Respiratory passages:** chronic hacking cough, asthma, convulsive bronchitis, frequent tonsillitis, swollen adenoids.

**Muscles and joints:** muscle pains, rheumatic joint pains and swollen joints.

**Bladder:** frequent urination, irritable bladder, enuresis and chronic infections of the urinary tract.

## The elimination diet – the way to freedom from symptoms

You won't be able to ignore the connection between your symptoms and incompatible foodstuffs if you suddenly get a skin rash after eating fish or strawberries.

Much more often, however, an allergy to a foodstuff is latent, i.e. there is no obvious connection between the food and the symptoms. The true state of affairs is further obscured by the complexity of the consequences, so that the sufferer, and often unfortunately, the doctor, gets the cause wrong.

**Self-testing with the elimination diet**

A food allergy can best be discovered by means of a trial elimination diet, which is based on the initial elimination of all food allergens for at least five days.

This can be achieved by fasting with no coffee, no tea, no fruit juice, just mineral water to drink, or by following a basal diet comprising only three or four foodstuffs that rarely involve incompatibility such as lamb, millet, rice, aubergines and thistle oil.

In most cases, a clear improvement or even a complete elimination of symptoms will be observed within five days – for example, for eczema both the reddening of the skin and the itch die away.

**Warning signals**

If foods are then eaten in succession as tests, the symptoms will return within anything from half an hour to several hours or, more rarely, one or two days, from the time that the first incompatible foodstuff was eaten. The skin rash of eczema worsens again, there is an attack of migraine or asthma, feelings of agitation or fear, hot flushes, digestive disorders or racing heartbeat, depending on the individual's syndrome.

The foods detected in this way should be eliminated from your diet with immediate effect, while compatible ones can of course be added to it.

● It's best to begin food trials with foods that rarely trigger an allergy. These are: rice (rice waffles), tapioca, millet, dried spelt, buckwheat, lamb, avocados, sweet potatoes, aubergines, broccoli, lettuce, cucumbers, courgettes, sugar peas, chick-peas, honeydew melons, mangoes, papayas, fresh figs, almonds which should be stewed shelled almonds from a health-food shop, coconut, maple syrup, sweeteners, thistle oil and sunflower oil.

● After these, choose foodstuffs from a group of medium compatibility, namely maize, spelt, sesame, sour-cream butter, sweet/sour cream, bio yoghurt, goat or sheep milk, beef, veal, chicken, turkey, trout, potatoes, green beans, beetroot, fennel, mangold, spinach, sweet apples, bananas, pears, dried sugar-cane juice, pear syrup and olive oil.

**Dangerous foods**

● Only at the end, and in the smallest doses, should you take the 'dangerous' foods, These are those that are frequently incompatible: wheat, rye, oats, barley, margarine, milk, cheese, eggs, pork, salt-water fish, fungi other than mushrooms, cauliflower, leguminous vegetables, carrots, red cabbage, white cabbage, savoy cabbage, leeks, onions, garlic, paprika, celery, parsley, sour apples, soft fruits, citrus fruits, grapes, nuts, sugar and blends of herb tea such as camomile, peppermint and fennel.

If you relieve your body from the stress of food allergens for a few months, it will recover to such an extent that you will find that many previously incompatible foods will gradually become compatible.

**No sugar, no pork**

Sugar and pork should always be avoided. In some circumstances it is also worth avoiding milk, milk products, eggs and citrus fruits.

Milk incompatibility is often present from birth. Even in infancy, it can be the cause of intestinal colic with screaming fits, flatulence, constipation or diarrhoea, and later susceptibility to infection, enlarged tonsils and recurrent inflammation of the middle ear.

A rotating or alternating diet is worthwhile for sufferers from food allergy, especially during the first year of therapy. Under it, the same food is only eaten on every fourth day. This helps to prevent the formation of new allergies and will make any existing ones disappear more quickly.

The success of the trial elimination diet depends on its being carried out strictly. For safety's sake, check with your doctor beforehand.

A five-day test using fasting or the basal diet, carried out as previously described, can be regarded as a spot check.

### Food allergy as a cause of other illnesses

It is suspected that a whole set of illnesses is actually caused by food allergy.

### Excess weight

**Excess weight can be due to a food allergy**

Excess weight is frequently due to food allergy. A large variety of foods can be incompatible: even coffee or sour apples, which contain few or no calories, can make you fat.

Here, again, the main villains are dairy products, wheat, a wide range of fruit and vegetables, sugar, and food additives. If allergens are eliminated from the diet, the pounds will mostly come off by themselves and you won't have to go on counting calories. The symptoms that frequently accompany excess weight – tiredness, lack of drive, irritability, restlessness, headaches, fear and depression – disappear at the same time.

**Are you addicted to the allergen?**

It won't exactly be easy for you to follow the described diet if you're addicted to your allergens. This frequently observed phenomenon is probably present if you have the feeling that you cannot live without chocolate, coffee, tea, cakes, bread, milk, yoghurt or apples.

Allergy researchers, therefore regard addiction to drugs, alcohol and nicotine as pure allergies to those substances.

Weight deficiency, too, can be a consequence of a food allergy. In such cases, dieting will cause a weight gain.

### Migraine

Powerful headaches, mostly on one side of the head and coming on like a fit, sometimes associated with sensitivity to light, indisposition and vomiting, spoil life for many sufferers.

A study by Dr J. Egger of Munich has shown that there is a food allergy, usually a hidden one, in more than 80 per cent of migraine cases. Here, too, then, the elimination diet is worth a trial.

### Gastrointestinal diseases

The consequences of a food incompatibility for the stomach and bowels can be so trivial that they don't get any further attention: a light-coloured, often pulpy stool, bloated stomach, and an unpleasant feeling of fullness.

But, chronic constipation or diarrhoea, too, can occur, all the way up to serious chronic illnesses like colitis ulcerosa, a chronic inflammation of the bowels typified by ulcers in the intestinal mucous membrane.

In Crohn's disease, too, which is accompanied by stomach pains, loss of weight, intestinal fistulas and diarrhoea, food allergy is important.

**Weight deficiency**

The intestinal flora is very often damaged and has to be rebuilt using appropriate preparations (page 38).

The possibility of a similar cause should also be considered in cases of gastric or duodenal ulcers or aphthous ulcers in the mouth.

### High or low blood pressure

In certain circumstances, making a test of the low-allergen diet can make the prolonged intake of an antihypertensive agent unnecessary, particularly where the combination of high blood pressure with another symptom listed above, leads to a suspicion of food allergy, for example migraine or excess weight.

**A doctor must exclude other causes**

Naturally, a doctor must first exclude other organic causes such as arteriosclerosis or renal disease. It is worth remembering that low blood pressure, too, is often associated with food allergy.

### Asthma

The possibility of a food allergy forming the basis for this chronic affliction is all too rarely considered (page 62).

Here, again, milk allergy plays the main role. The food incompatibility is almost invariably hidden, only being disclosed by the elimination diet and test meals.

If milk has been omitted for some time a sip of milk can trigger an asthma attack, although usually other foods are involved as well.

In the case of asthma you will need to seek expert medical guidance as supervision is invariably necessary in the case of any prescribed treatment.

## Rheumatic joint complaints

A very frequent sign of food allergy is pains in the joints and muscles – even children may suffer from them.

**Dietary change**

A change of diet often brings success in cases of chronic rheumatism and arthritis, but an initial two to three week fast is advisable here. After that you should perform the test and avoid food allergens. Instead, you should eat base-rich raw food as far as you can. It is precisely in the case of rheumatic joint complaints that hyperacidification of the body tissue often occurs, caused in particular by animal protein such as meat, fish and eggs, but also by concentrated 'empty' carbohydrates such as sugar, white flour and starch.

Where joints have already been ruined, however, an alleviation of the pain can often still be attained. Primary chronic polyarthritis (the inflammation of several joints that can occur following an angina) has different origins and therefore the advice given above does not apply to this condition.

## Susceptibility to infection

A chronic tendency to infections such as sinusitis, bronchitis, tonsillitis, inflammation of the middle ear or colds, is often caused by a food allergy. This applies particularly in the case of small children, who are frequently unwell. The cause in many cases is a hereditary milk allergy. Once the allergens are removed from their food, their state of health usually improves markedly.

**Bedwetting**

The administration of doses of antibiotics can worsen the situation by intensifying the disruption of the intestinal flora that already exists (page 38). This also applies to recurrent inflammation of the bladder. Like bedwetting, this is often a consequence and expression of a food allergy and it is only cured when all the food allergens have been eliminated from the diet.

### Hay fever

Diet is the key treatment

Here too, the basis is often a food incompatibility on to which the pollen allergy is then 'grafted'. If you stick to the diet, therefore, even the plague of hay fever can sometimes be alleviated (page 44).

Sometimes it is enough just to eliminate milk during the hay-fever season.

### Eczema

As already mentioned, eczema is often based on food allergy. The skin often quickly improves if the food allergens are eliminated and promptly worsens again if an incompatible food is eaten. In contrast to other syndromes, it is easy to spot both positive and negative reactions simply by seeing how an affected persons skin reacts.

### Nettle rash (urticaria)

In this illness, itching skin spots can suddenly form, then quickly lose intensity, only to reappear somewhere else.

In children especially

The cause, particularly in children, is often a vegetable allergen with which the skin has come into contact, an insect sting or more rarely pollen, dust, chemicals (colourants, preservatives, foods) or components of creams, oils, detergents and fruit sprays.

Internal causes of nettle rash also include bacteria, viruses and fungi.

It is important here to proceed like a criminologist in order to find out the cause and eliminate it, if possible.

Therapeutically, all the measures recommended above are indicated if they reduce your tendency to allergy and improve your general physical condition.

In any case, it is worth trying out the test diet in order to exclude a food allergy.

### Contact allergy

Skin contact with an allergen mostly leads to inflammatory reddening and itching of the area involved within 24-48 hours. Typically, such eczema appears on the ear lobes because of earrings containing nickel, in the area of the navel because of a stud on your jeans, or under your wristwatch.

Apart from nickel, there is a wide variety of chemicals involved – including industrial ones. Here is a selection of jobs and the substances they may be exposed to.

Typical work-related allergens

Nurses: disinfectants and medicines; bakers: citron oil, bitter almond oil, yeast and benzoic acid; hairdressers: hair dyes, perm solutions and perfumes; farmers: plant protection products and artificial fertilizers; office and printshop workers: ink, tracing paper, printing inks, adhesives and felt-tipped pens; metalworkers: oils, lubricants and rust inhibitors; housewives: detergents, cleaning agents, floor wax and rubber, plus cosmetics, hygiene products and much more besides.

Here too, it is a matter of identifying the incompatible substances by c ritical observation or by performing the appropriate tests — for example the linen-patch test, (see page 16) — and avoiding them in future. In serious cases, this may of course mean a change of occupation.

Sometimes the underlying cause of contact eczema is an allergy to foods such as milk or eggs and the condition improves when the diet is corrected.

Contact dermatitis is abetted by skin damage. As a preventive measure, avoid all contact with chemicals (including rubber and plastic gloves), don't use soap containing alkalis that damage the skin's acidic coating, and apply lotion frequently.

## Psoriasis

The external disfigurement of round, red foci, mostly covered with silvery flakes, on the arms and legs and often on the back, buttocks and head, puts heavy psychological stress on most sufferers. This can often cause more distress to the sufferer than the condition itself.

**A mental strain**

There is often a connection with food incompatibility here. Herbs, alcohol, sweets and sugar make things worse. Occasionally there is an improvement if these substances are removed from the diet. Otherwise, the elimination diet (see page 64) is certainly worth trying in an attempt to help to identify the possible cause. Treatment with fumaric acid in the form of capsules, ointment or lotion often has a beneficial and supportive effect.

### Hyperkinetic syndrome (hyperactivity in children)

The number of children who are so agitated they can't sit still, is growing all the time.

Such children rub everyone up the wrong way. They're considered badly brought up, are disruptive in school, can't concentrate and are often weak in reading, spelling and mathematics. During puberty they may be conspicuous for aggression and truancy and be subject to an above-average risk of addiction.

The Hyperactive Children's Support Group (see address on page 103) is able to supply information to help problems related to hyperactivity and allergy. Parents in the 'Hyperactive Child Study Group' a German research group, have discovered that children's symptoms can often be **Elimination** radically alleviated within one or two weeks by a low-**diet** allergen diet, free from phosphates and other food additives. The vast majority of children that were treated, became far less hyperactive and much better balanced.

This is reason enough to carry out a trial of the elimination diet with such children before reaching for such drastic remedies as Ritalin or amphetamine.

There's far too little realization that quite 'normal' foods, **Triggered by** and the food additives used everywhere these days, can be **food** incompatible and seriously disrupt our mental equilibrium. They can be to blame for irritability, aggression, nervousness, agitation, lack of concentration, resignation, weariness, lack of drive and serious depression. Those affected complain of groundless states of anxiety and panic.

It's worth considering the possibility of a food allergy first before spending years taking psychopharmaceuticals. The possible connection between depression and mercury poisoning from amalgam fillings, formaldehyde and wood preservatives (page 26) have already been referred to. Even convulsions (epileptic attacks) can occur because of food allergy.

# Natural treatments

There are many natural healing options that enable a doctor to strengthen the endogenous regulatory and defensive system. However, it is not possible to go into them all here. Essentially the therapies that can be effective in allergic disorders involve avoidence of the allergen, desensitization techniques (page 49) and a variety of approaches to strengthen the body's resistance to allergens. This can involve detoxification techniques such as those used by naturopaths, homeopathy, vitamin and mineral supplementation as well as a variety of physiological techniques that may enhance the body's healing abilities.

**Supportive therapies**

## Homeopathy

No method of natural healing is so strongly disputed as homeopathy. Again and again it is disparaged as charlatanism – mainly by people who have never studied it in detail. By contrast, homeopathic doctors and patients keep reporting impressive successes that cannot be written off as imaginary, especially since veterinary surgeons can show a similar catalogue of success. It is impossible to say homeopathy is 'all in the mind' when it cures a horse.

This healing method was established by Samuel Hahnemann (1755-1843), a German doctor and scientist. By experimenting on himself he discovered that taking quinine, then widely used for treating malaria, would cause the symptoms of malaria to appear in a healthy person. From this and other experiments, he derived the similarity rule as the basis of homeopathy.

This rule states that like is cured with like. In the event of illness, therefore, medicine is used that, tested on a healthy person, produces the same symptoms as those displayed by the patient.

**'Like cures like'**

Substances of animal, vegetable or mineral origin (for example spider venom) serve as the basis for homeopathic preparations. They are diluted and shaken according to quite specific rules. It struck Hahnemann that their effect was substantially increased in the now proverbial 'homeopathic doses', although these were so heavily diluted as not to contain a single molecule of the original substance.

**Made from natural substances**

As a rule, homeopathic remedies are named from their basic substance, for example lycopodium (club moss), nux vomica, phosphorus, etc. The name of the preparation is followed by the power, i.e. the nature and frequency of the dilution and shaking processes.

D6, for example, means that the relevant substance was diluted and shaken a total of six times, starting with a dilution of 1:10 (D = decimal power). This allows a dilution of 1:1 to be attained. The process is called 'potentiation'.

It is these dilutions that doubters and critics are always questioning: 'pure water' can't do anything, they say. But the latest findings of modern physics indicate that what we are dealing with are energy effects, and the approximate explanation for them is that the 'information' in the substance has been transferred to the solvent and it is the latter, not the former, that effects the healing.

**Energy effects**

The art of the homeopathic doctor consists of finding out the appropriate remedy for each individual patient. To do this he is guided not only by the patient's symptoms, but also by the special features of his personality. He determines these by questioning the patient comprehensively about his preferences and aversions, habits and characteristics. Such constitutional agent, which is specially adapted to the patient's personality, has a profound effect not only on physical complaints but also on factors in the mental and spiritual domain.

**Long term treatment**

Determining the constitutional agent is a very time-consuming process; it usually can't be covered by a health insurance, but has to be paid for by the patient himself. In certain cases, the process can be shortened and a simplification can be achieved by prescribing a complex agent, a mixture of a few homeopathic preparations. This doesn't require the precise selection that is entailed in the selection of individual remedies. Such complex agents have familiar names and are suitable for 'narrow-gauge' use for acute states of ill health such as colds.

However, even homeopathy has its limits where many chronic afflictions (cancer, dangerous infections, hormone deficiencies or diabetes) are concerned.

In the case of allergies, a trial is always worthwhile, especially with a constitutional agent that has already healed many allergies without the illness reappearing later. But patience is required here. Since 'primary immune responses' can sometimes occur, the treatment should be left to an experienced homeopath.

**Patience is required**

If you have a food allergy and you want try the elimination diet in order to test the compatibility of different foods (page 64) you should not take homeopathic remedies at the same time, because possible reactions to the medicines and incompatibility reactions to foods, will mask each other.

**Important!**

### Acupuncture

An extremely wide range of disturbances to health can be influenced for the good by stimulating certain points on the body. This was first observed more than 2,000 years ago by the Chinese, who developed a system of rules on the subject. Their adherence to these rules over such a prolonged period is testimony to the indisputable results attained by acupuncture.

**Stimulated with needles**

Like homeopathy it also works on animals, so the lay view that it's all in the mind collapses here, too.

The acupuncture points can be stimulated with needles (the commonest method), a laser beam, heat or massage (acupressure). The laser beam is quite painless – ideal for children. Irradiation of the acupuncture points for 15-30 seconds yields the same results as the use of needles.

Migraine, sinusitis, trigeminal neuralgia, bedwetting, trouble with the locomotor system such as lumbago, shoulder and neck pains are well attested areas of application. This method works on allergies, too. In hay fever and eczema it eases the symptoms.

An acupuncture sequence should always be carried out in cases of asthma because it lends support to other therapeutic applications, which are indispensable in a chronic affliction like this.

Ear acupuncture: all the regions of the body, from top to toe, are 'depicted' on a small scale in the outer ear. Effective treatment can often be given with needles or a painless laser beam via these points.

### Electro-acupuncture

Dr Reinhard Voll developed this special form of acupuncture in the 1950s. Above and beyond this, it is to his credit that, in addition to the points already known from Chinese acupuncture, he discovered a further whole series of new ones and made connections between these and internal organs and tissues.

Using a purpose-made appliance, in broad terms the electrical resistance of the skin is measured at various acupuncture points. This provides information about the energy state of the associated organs. If the skin's resistance is high, an inflammation or irritation is present. If it is low, this is a sign of a debilitated condition.

**Diagnosis can be made**

So it is possible to use these types of electro-acupuncture techniques to arrive at a diagnosis, and frequently before clinical symptoms have fully formed or findings can be arrived at in a pathological laboratory. Clearly, therapy can be much more successful at this early stage than later, when irreparable organic damage may have developed.

The skin's conductivity also gives an indication of what medicine may help. If, for example, a homeopathic agent is introduced into the oscillatory circuit of the equipment and an unhealthy reading returns to normal, the doctor giving treatment knows that the right remedy has been found. The remedies used in academic medicine can be tested in the same way.

It's of particular importance these days that the Voll method of electro-acupuncture enables doctors to detect stresses imposed on the body by poisons, for example pesticides, insecticides, formaldehyde, and heavy metals like cadmium, lead and mercury (dental fillings). Such materials can be extracted from the body using certain homeopathic dilutions of the substance involved. The same is true for poisons that have been accumulated in the body after an earlier illness, which may have occurred years or even decades before.

**Good for allergic illness**

A further advantage of electro-acupuncture is the possibility it affords of testing seats of disease in the teeth, tonsils, caecum (blind gut) and other organs via the acupuncture points. For allergy sufferers it's possible to detect allergens this way, especially incompatible foods.

The reliability of testing and the success of treatment both depend on the therapist's skill. Voll's techniques have been further developed by a number of other authorities and now form part of a broad group of medicine testing and diagnostic procedures which are best grouped under the general heading of 'functional medicine'.

### Foot reflexology
Parts of our bodies and all our organs are reflected in firmly defined areas on the soles of our feet. Diseased organs can be detected when there is pain in the corresponding area. If the latter is massaged, using the sole of the foot like a control panel, profound effects can be achieved.
- The excretory organs (skin, kidneys, bowels and respiratory passages) are stimulated.
- Headaches and stomach pains are reduced, and renal or intestinal colic is interrupted.
- The vegetative nervous system is harmonized, energy is increased and sleeplessness is eased.

**Effective in many illnesses**

Because it stimulates all bodily functions, foot reflexology is also reliable in cases of allergy.

It is important to go to a qualified reflexologist as mishandling can easily cause damage, but specially trained therapists can obtain amazing results.
A similar effect is obtained with a cure using Schiele

circulatory equipment. This is a footbath with an electric heater underneath that heats it up to 35 to 45°C in steps, depending on tolerance. During this bath, all areas of the sole of the foot are activated by the increasing warmth.

Various supplements can be added to the water. The footbath can have amazing effects on a variety of complaints, such as migraine, chronic digestive disorders, inflammation of the bladder, complaints of the lower abdomen and sleeplessness. With allergies, too, the equipment, which can be rented, is recommended for giving general assistance.

*The footbath can work on a variety of compaints*

### Bioresonance therapy

A development is at hand for which the often misused word 'sensational' can happily be used.

Whereas chemistry has been the godfather of previous forms of therapy, biophysical methods will play an ever greater role in the medicine of the future. Extremely fine signals, too weak for the human senses to detect, control the processes going on in our bodies. If we are thoroughly healthy, harmonic oscillations occur but, if we are sick, they are mixed with diseased, inharmonious oscillations.

*Diagnostic procedure*

Modern research has shown these connections to be fascinating. Professor C. W. Smith of Salford University exposed 150 volunteer patients at a London allergy clinic to a weak alternating voltage at various frequencies. One of these guinea-pigs was a young woman who habitually reacted to her allergen with severe gait problems, which meant she could only move around with difficulty.

It was possible to induce exactly the same symptoms by transmitting electromagnetic waves at a frequency of 2.5 hertz from a sinusoidal oscillator at a distance of 3m, using a wire 1.5m long as an antenna. This drastic effect was achieved using an extremely weak current. The voltage at the antenna was only 1 volt and at the patient's position this was too low to be measured. When Professor Smith changed the frequency to 154 hertz, he immediately erased the gait problems: the patient was once more able to walk.

*Profound effects*

But even more astonishing, Professor Smith then placed

a small tub of water near the oscillator and treated this with the 'healing' (neutralizing) frequency. When he merely put this in the patient's hand, her gait problems were just as immediately erased.

All this makes it easier to understand why high homeopathic powers (page 73) can have an effect even when not a single molecule of the original substance is present. The information, the biophysical signal, operates even in the absence of material.

This experiment using low voltages and different frequencies, which can mimic or erase the symptoms of allergy for each patient, gives grounds for supposing that illnesses are associated with a specific energy wave and can be healed by a different energy wave.

**Specific energy waves**

Ten years ago, Dr Franz Morell introduced the Mora principle into therapy. Via electrodes on the hands and feet, oscillations on the surface of the patient's skin are detected and led to a device in which the unhealthy energies are transformed into their opposites, i.e. they are cancelled, while the harmonic oscillations of the patient are strengthened. The patient's intrinsic oscillations are fed back through a cable as a therapeutic signal to support the endogenous regulatory system.

Further development has yielded an appliance which, under automatic control, supplies the body with a band of various frequencies from which the body 'picks out' its 'healing' frequency. The other frequencies have no effect and are swept through at high speed but the organism reacts to them more slowly.

**Healing frequencies**

Lykotronic therapy works in a similar way and, by harmonizing the body's energy centres (chakras), operates very successfully using the body's endogenous oscillations.

The area of application of bioresonance therapy is as large as the range of illnesses. It is well proven in the case of allergies such as asthma, hay fever and eczema.

Using the diagnostic section of the equipment and the principle of electro-acupuncture (see page 76), trained therapists can also test for food incompatibilities.

### Phototherapy

The favourable effect of coloured light on a number of illnesses has long been known. A disadvantage hitherto has been the lengthy treatment time involved. But modern electronics have brought about a change here.

Depending on requirements, a colour apparatus injects colours (red, orange, yellow, green, blue and violet) into the body via a hand-held probe or at acupuncture points. A few minutes are enough.

Therapy using coloured light is well attested for nervousness, digestive disorders, allergies, asthma and other illnesses. It also supplements other natural healing methods.Phototherapy can be provided through a variety of different pieces of equipment available both in the UK and in Germany.

**Therapy using coloured lights**

### Phytotherapy

Nature is one large chemist shop. Modern medicine is continually rediscovering the multiple effects of medicinal plants that had been forgotten in the light of modern discoveries. The pharmaceutical industry is devoting ever more intensive efforts into research on the agents that are contained in every plant.

It's the interaction of all the contents that makes up the typical effect of a medicinal plant. If a single substance is isolated, for example the cardiac medicine digitalis from purple foxglove, the effect can be quite different from that of a synthesized version.

In everyday infections such as influenza, coughing, or gastrointestinal complaints, medicinal plants can perform a useful service by supporting the organism in a gentle way, so that more powerful remedies can be avoided.

**Supporting the organism in gentle ways**

An allergy sufferer above all should be careful to give his body as few chemicals as possible for 'digestion'. But he must also realize that he could also react allergically to natural remedies such as medicinal plants. Despite their healing effect, camomile, fennel, St John's wort, peppermint and marigold are sometimes incompatible and should therefore be used with caution.

## Treatment using minerals and trace elements

These substances, which we normally obtain from our food, are of decisive importance for our metabolic processes.

Out of the large number of vital materials, the most important are: calcium, chromium, potassium, copper, magnesium, iron, manganese, sodium, phosphorus, selenium, silicium and zinc.

There are several reasons why in our industrial society many people have a deficiency of minerals and trace elements.

● Reduced intake: intensive farming has leached out our soils, artificial fertilizers have dislocated the natural relationships between the minerals in the soil, and acid rain has caused some plants to take up too few minerals.

On top of this, we eat processed foods and too few full-grain products, vegetables and salads, which are the main sources of important minerals and trace elements. White flour and sugar even rob us of these important substances, which are used up in processing these 'empty carbohydrates'.

**Deficient in important substances**

● Defective resorption: if the power of our digestive system is impaired by an alteration of our intestinal milieu on account of unhealthy eating, or if the mucous membrane is irritated and inflamed because we've eaten food allergens, the minerals in the food can't be sufficiently absorbed.

● Environmental pollution: because of the effects of the heavy metals to which we are exposed nowadays, such as mercury, cadmium and lead, our mineral budget can become dislocated, which in turn leads to deficiency phenomena.

The consequences of mineral and trace-element deficiency are as follows:

● Calcium deficiency: muscle cramps, nervousness, loss of bone calcium and arthritis;

● Magnesium deficiency: headaches, drowsiness, stomach upsets, depression, restlessness, anxiety states, calf cramps, irregular heartbeat, stomach cramps and circulatory disorders;

**Symptoms of mineral deficiency**

● Zinc deficiency: susceptibility to infection, delayed healing of wounds, disturbed concentration and delayed growth and sexual maturation;

● Selenium deficiency: Keshan disease (a serious cardiac illness) and increased susceptibility to cancer. Most important of all, selenium gives protection from the effects of environmental poisons such as cadmium, lead and mercury. Selenium, in combination with vitamins and minerals, is contained in antioxidant preparations. The latter protect us from highly poisonous substances (free radicals) that form in our bodies because of environmental pollution.

**Analysis of hair minerals**

Subject to a few caveats, a deficiency of minerals and trace elements can be investigated by an analysis of hair minerals. Although blood tests can sometimes be helpful, relationships in the blood are subject to frequent variation, whereas the substances that are tested in our hair remain constant.

Stress from heavy metals can also be detected by this means. Allergy sufferers, especially, will find a hair-mineral analysis worthwhile, since many of them display a deficiency of calcium, magnesium, zinc, manganese and selenium, and a surplus of mercury, lead and cadmium. Compensatory measures can have a favourable effect on the allergy, but should be carried out by a doctor who is experienced in this kind of treatment.

You can safely take a power cocktail cure on your own initiative. This is a preparation of vital substances consisting of wheat, wild barley and two species of algae. The cocktail will detoxify the body with its chlorophyll content, and supply it with a natural blend of numerous vitamins, trace elements and enzymes.

**Make your own power cocktail**

### Enzyme therapy

Our metabolic and digestive functions are controlled by proteins, the enzymes, which act like the sparks from a car ignition. They are often blocked by the manifold effects of the poisons we are exposed to nowadays. This in turn leads to defective digestion and disturbances in the biochemical processes from which we obtain energy and materials for the construction of bodily substance from our food.

**Defective digestion**

Allergies are often combined with digestive enzyme deficiency and your doctor may recommend that you take an appropriate digestive enzyme preparation for a few weeks.

### Provocative and neutralization testing

The intradermal provocative and neutralization test is a method developed in the USA for simultaneously testing for and treating allergies, particularly allergies to foods and chemicals. Allergens are diluted with salt water on a 1:5 basis and are made up into a set of serially diluted containers, each with progressively less allergen than the first. These dilutions are then injected into a weal in the skin of the upper arm. If the weal increases in size by 2mm or more within ten minutes, an incompatibility exists. Other symptoms which confirm this are sweating, headache, indisposition, stomach pains, exhaustion and depression.

Various dilutions of the allergen are injected and the patient is observed until the dose is identified where the weal ceases to grow and symptoms disappear. This dilution is then termed the 'neutralizing dose'. The patient then has regular injections of the neutralizing dose.

After a period of time, the incompatibility recedes and the patient can more easily tolerate the allergen concerned. During the testing process, however, there are occasionally reactions. The method is costly in both time and money, and is used in only a few places.

**Costly in both time and money**

There is another method, that is the same in principle but technically different, which allows pollen, chemicals and medicines to be tested and therapeutic dilutions to be discovered (see page 49).

### Health through self-help

To be healthy you have to spend time taking care of your body. To start with you need to be honest with yourself: do you eat too much of all the wrong things, drink alcohol, smoke cigarettes and get too little fresh air, take too little exercise and have too little sleep?

Be honest
with
yourself
Your body will put up with all these things for quite a time, with just a few grumbles at first – then suddenly, in the form of token strikes and downright sickness, it will bring you the bill.

This picture is especially true for allergies. Although an allergic illness is frequently based on hereditary predisposition, it is a proven fact that these hereditary factors often do not have any effect while the affected person remains in top condition, mentally and physically.

Of course natural healing has a part to play in helping you to be healthy, but there are many things that you personally can do to get yourself into tip-top condition.

### You are what you eat

It is astonishing the profound effect a change of diet can make to a large number of illnesses, especially allergies.

To supply your body with all the necessary vitamins, minerals and trace elements it is very important to follow the wholefoods principle. This means that you should, as far as is possible, eat only wholefoods.

These are the implications for your menu:

● Get rid of tinned foods, ready-prepared meals and convenient packaged foods, and get back to fresh, home prepared meals, raw for preference.   Change your diet

● Get rid of white flour, white bread, white rolls, cakes, biscuits, puddings and sweets, replacing them with wholemeal bread and full-grain products and, most important of all, fresh full-grain muesli in the morning that you made yourself the previous evening from cereals which you soaked overnight. You can finish it off according to taste with some yoghurt, cream, honey, nuts and seasonal fruit.

● Before your midday meal eat a good portion of salad, include grated carrots, fennel, cucumber, tomatoes, radishes, Jerusalem artichokes and, if you like, apples, a few segments of orange, pineapple and raisins, dressed with sour cream, yoghurt or a good cold pressed oil.

● Instead of eating peeled potatoes boiled in salt water, eat potatoes boiled in their skins. Include some dried spelt,

buckwheat and millet in your menu frequently.
● Eat little or no meat; eat more vegetables instead, carefully steamed, rather than boiled.
● Eat unpolished rice instead of the polished variety and noodles made from wholemeal rather than white flour.
● Instead of putting jam, honey or sausage on your bread, use cress, chives, quark, slices of cucumber or banana, or raspberry jelly.
● Don't sweeten your food with sugar but, if something really must be sweetened, use pear syrup, dried sugar-cane juice or a good maple syrup.

The shelves of the bookshops are groaning under the wide range of cookery books devoted to wholemeal food. In them you will find recipes to suit every taste. Look through them and you will discover that to be healthy you don't have to put tasteless grains and greens on the table. There are hundreds of tasty recipes to choose from if you decide to introduce a new healthy regime into your life and that of your family.

**Tasty recipes**

A useful tip: The less you say about a new dish you are serving being 'particularly healthy', the less likelihood there is of your partner or children refusing to eat it!

## Compatible food combinations

We often overload our digestive systems by eating too much and jumbling different foods together. There is a well proven principle which is usually helpful: don't overfill your plate, and chew every bite at least 30 times. If you don't gobble your food, you will feel full sooner and eat less.

A particularly effective approach, especially if your pancreas has been damaged by malnourishment, is the Hay method of combining compatible foods (named after an American, Dr Howard Hay).

The Hay diet states that protein and sour fruits need to be digested in an acid solution while starch and sugar, on the other hand, being carbohydrates, need a basic solution. For that reason, you should never eat the two food groups together at one meal: meat goes with vegetables, but never with potatoes, noodles or rice.

The Hay diet    Many people who have tried this diet have reported that their excess weight, diabetes, sore joints and digestive complaints have greatly improved and that they don't feel so tired after meals as they used to do.

Even if it means changing your eating habits, you should give this method your attention.

### Fasting

The profound effect a fast has on the body, and on moods, has been known for years. If our organs are released for a while from the daily effort of digestion, they diligently set about spring-cleaning themselves and eliminating accumulated waste products.

A precondition for a full fasting cure is that the kidneys and the liver are working well so that they are actually able to cope with eliminating all the waste products, otherwise, auto-intoxication may occur. So, before you start fasting it is a good idea to ask your doctor for his advice.

**Ask your doctor for advice**

### Things you need to know about fasting

● You will experience hunger at first but this will be temporary; you can easily overcome it by drinking a lot of liquids.

● An additional intake of liquids (2-3 litres a day) is absolutely necessary for flushing you out: herbal tea, uncarbonated mineral water or spring water are best.

● You should also have a daily enema to cleanse the bowels, a daily liver compress and plenty of exercise in the fresh air.

● The minimum fasting period is seven days, but two or even three weeks is better.

● It is best to fast while you are on holiday. People whose health is not absolutely sound should always put themselves in the care of a doctor. If you wish to fast on your own, make sure that you have obtained all the information you require beforehand by doing the relevant reading so that you do not make mistakes and do yourself more harm than good.

Caution is required in the case of people who have had

problems with heavy metals such as lead, mercury or cadmium, or from wood preservatives. Because of heavy environmental pollution, many people are affected without knowing it these days (page 26). During a fast these poisons, which have accumulated in the fatty tissue of the body, are suddenly released into the system. Damage will be done if, because of defective functioning of the liver or a kidney, or an insufficient intake of fluid, these are not flushed out.

**Caution may be required**

This is the reason why people who fast do not always feel like a million dollars, despite the claim that is frequently made. Another contributing factor is that a profound metabolic change-over is involved during fasts. Sometimes fasting may cause a mineral deficiency, for example, of magnesium. This would have to be remedied by taking an appropriate preparation, such as Basica.

In all cases it is important not to start a fasting cure without some preparation. Begin preparing your body by eating less food and ensuring any food you do eat is raw and rich in vital substances, such as minerals and vitamins. Partial fasting methods are less drastic and therefore gentler.

**Fasting may cause a mineral deficiency**

The Mayr cure: you only eat dry rolls and you must chew small bites until there is nothing left in your mouth. Drink milk from a teaspoon along with the rolls. Great care is devoted to a sophisticated method of stomach massage, intended to activate the bowel.

The Mayr cure is a good alternative for people who don't want to go through a full fast. From a doctor's point of view, it can be highly recommended. But patients who suffer from a wheat or milk allergy can follow this cure only in a modified form. This should be borne in mind by anyone who feels worse instead of better during the cure.

The fruit-juice cure: in connection with the fruit-juice cure, you must remember that you could have an allergy to a particular fruit juice, or to one of the vegetables in the vegetable broth, or to the yeast that is added for enrichment. Flatulence and feelings of satiation are grounds for suspicion.

Fruit-juice cure

The 600-calorie diet: this diet consists of fruit, raw salads, vegetables, potatoes, quark and a cold-pressed oil such as thistle oil. You shouldn't use any salt, but you do need to drink a lot of liquid.

Although you won't lose a lot of weight on this diet, the body will be supplied with sufficient protein and vital substances so you can go on working without hindrance.

### Your body – use it or lose it

The second big maltreatment that we inflict on our body is to give it insufficient exercise and fresh air. You should exercise every day if possible, or alternatively at least three times a week, for a minimum of 20 minutes to start with, gradually building up the time as you become fitter.

To walk around the block every evening is certainly better than doing nothing, but you really need to increase your heart-rate for at least ten minutes each day.

Jogging is very popular nowadays, but it has the disadvantage that it is rather a one-sided form of exercise and it leads to overexertion and imposes a not insubstantial load on the joints.

Increase your heart-rate

From a medical standpoint, doing morning exercises at an open window is preferable since, if you use a mixed exercise programme, all your muscle groups will be called upon. There is a wide range of records and cassettes giving expert instruction, as well as lively music which will help you turn your obligatory morning exercises into fun.

Another, more refined, way of doing a great deal for your body without too much exertion is jumping on a mini trampoline. The amazing effect is based on the alternation of weightlessness while jumping and the gentle springing on landing, which imposes exercise on a lymphatic system that may have been overstressed by waste products and become sluggish. This has been reported as having favourable effects on the most varied complaints – from migraine to back pains.

Jump on a mini trampoline

Five minutes, three times a day, is enough at the beginning. Later you can work up to 15 minutes, twice daily (morning and evening). Try putting some lively music on to

**Exercise for people who are no good at sport**

help get you going in the morning and help you wind down in the evening. This kind of training is ideal for people who are no good at sport but still want to keep fit.

You should also treat yourself to an extended walk as often as you can. This should include bursts in which you shift to an easy trot, or at least go as fast as you can. Strolling along slowly, without any great effort, does not do you a lot of good.

## How to stimulate your circulation

The fact that short, sharp shocks with cold water stimulate the circulation and vegetative system, and can have a benign influence on even serious illnesses was put to the test last century by Father Kneipp, of Wrishofen, on his numerous patients. His methods – baths, infusions and compresses – are described in many books. These are a few of his methods that are easily applied but very effective:

### Paddling

**Cold water**

Run cold water into the bath until it is level with the middle of your lower leg, and paddle around in it as though picking your way very gingerly, lifting each leg in turn right out of the water.

Do this for 1-2 minutes. If you feel cold, stop immediately. Never enter the water with cold feet. Afterwards, just wipe the water off quickly with your hands and let your feet dry off under the bedclothes or in the open air, keeping them moving.

**Caution may be required**

### Brush massage

Massage with a dry brush is a well proven supplement to paddling. Using a soft handbrush, a massage band or a massage glove, first brush the legs from bottom to top, then do the trunk up to the heart, the arms from hand to shoulder, and finally the neck and back. Use powerful strokes that leave the skin slightly reddened and feeling pleasantly warm.This is easy and hardly takes any time so everybody can enjoy its far-reaching and beneficial effects.

### Cold-water rub-down

This water application is especially designed to strengthen the sexual organs, the bladder and the bowels.

Standing over a basin or bidet, give yourself a cold-water rub-down twice weekly using a rough flannel. Rub the lower abdomen and the sexual organs firmly but gently with cold water. Once you have got used to the cold water, try giving yourself a rub-down in a cold bath, twice a week.

**Long-lasting effects**

You will find that after each session you are left with a long-lasting warm glow and a feeling of invigorated freshness and enhanced vitality. This is due to the strengthening and harmonization of the vegetative nervous system.

### How to stimulate elimination via the skin

Apart from the kidneys and bowels, the skin is our greatest and most important excretory organ. Through it we get rid of metabolic products that would otherwise burden down our body.

In the past, before technology relieved us of heavy work, most people literally earned their bread by the sweat of their brow. Large quantities of poisons were excreted together with the sweat. Nowadays machines do most of the hard manual work so we have to try to detoxify our bodies in some other way.

### Saunas

A regular trip to the sauna is a well-proven method of detoxification. The alternate warming and cooling of the body in a pool, or under a cold shower, causes metabolic wastes to be exuded. The associated hardening effect makes the body much less liable to infection.

Even for allergy sufferers, a sauna is highly recommended. Of course, eczema patients in the acutest stage must be careful because the warmth and sweating can cause intensification of the itching. In general, however, saunas are considered helpful to the sufferers of skin diseases because they make the skin feel so clean and soft afterwards.

**Well-proven method**

### Long baths

This bath, too, has a profound and purifying effect on the system and drives poisons out of the body fluids. Some doctors in the USA have enthusiastically reported on the enlivening effect of a long bath. They say that they make their patients feel as though they could 'tear trees out by the roots'.

*Enlivening effect*

But you need to have plenty of time for this type of bath. The recommended period you should spend in the bath is three hours, five is better and, optimally, you should stay in for eight hours.

The water, which should reach up to your throat, must be kept at a constant 37°C (the temperature of your blood) by an inflow of warm water. Lower temperatures cause undesirable shivering, while higher ones overload the circulation. The effect is enhanced if you add a cupful of vinegar to the bath water.

*Keep water at a constant temperature*

In cases of rheumatism and gout the addition of 3-4 lbs of Epsom salts after five hours in the bath is recommended, followed by a further half-hour in the bath, to achieve an impressive improvement in the joints.

The day before the bath, you should fast or eat only fruit or a little raw food. During the bath, you should only drink fruit or vegetable juice. Immediately before getting into the bath you should give yourself an enema, as a sort of preliminary internal cleansing. You will need to rest for about an hour after the bath.

*Drink only fruit or vegetable juice*

People say that after 25 baths, you will feel 25 years younger. The fact that, after five hours, the water has a yellowish tinge (even if you're a fanatic about your personal hygiene) and is beginning to have an unpleasant smell is sufficient evidence that waste products and pollutants are being flushed out of the uttermost depths of our bodies.

Perhaps some rainy weekend you'd like to do something for your health and try a long bath. Lay a large folded towel on the bottom of the bath, set up a radio or TV in the bathroom or put some books on an improvised shelf, and relax in the warm water.

Patients with cardiovascular problems or serious

illnesses should not try out the long bath without first taking medical advice.

It is important to remember too that not everyone can immediately stand being in a long bath for the recommended period of three hours, so it is a good idea to increase your bathing time gradually: one hour for the first bath, two for the second, and so on.

## Long showers

For this shower you will need a recirculating pump (in order to save hot water), a special shower head and a holder for it. Lie in the bath once or twice a week and be showered with water at 41°C. The shower is hand-controlled so that every part of the body can get the benefit.

Several factors work in combination here: as in the long bath, metabolic residues are flushed out of the body. Then there is a soft massage effect because of the pressure from the small water-jets. Oxygen, drawn out of the air by the falling water, is probably of additional benefit to the body, so is the weak electric charge that results when hot water flows through cool air.

**Every part of the body gets the benefit**

The enlivening and stimulating effect, like that of a long bath, is often compared to a true fountain of youth.

## Rest and recuperation

Since more and more of our work is being taken over by technological advances these days, and many of us only work a 35-hour week, it is usually our own fault if we complain of stress and strain.

**Plan your holiday carefully**

Insufficient self-organization is one of our most frequent faults. Just think for a moment about changes you could make in your personal and working life. Make sure you don't burden your leisure time with yet more stress. Plan to take your holiday at a time and in an area that, by its climate alone, contributes to your health. This means beside the sea, or up in the hills or the mountains.

Put together your own tailor-made health programme for this period. If you really want to relax and recuperate your holiday should be for at least three weeks or more.

### Emotional balance – the basis of good health

Pessimism, negative thoughts and moping are bad for the health. They can actually cause various illnesses or make them persist. It's been scientifically proven that a negative attitude to life not only has a similarly negative effect on our intestinal bacteria and the coagulation of our blood, it also weakens our immune system. This in turn opens the door to every possible illness – starting with susceptibility to infection and moving on through allergies, all the way up to cancer. Knowing this should be reason enough to do something, not just for our bodies but also for our emotional balance.

**Negative thoughts are bad for our health**

No person's life is a continuous bed of roses. We all have to overcome strokes of fate such as the death and illness of those close to us, painful break ups and partings, disillusionment, setbacks at work, unemployment – not to mention the many little everyday irritations.

Yet there are many people who have had to cope with heavy emotional burdens who have still been able to retain a cheerful outlook. They usually have a firm foothold in terms of faith – though the church community may have little to do with this. What counts is their feeling of being guided by a higher power and the certainty that everything, even affliction, sickness and the blows of fate, has a meaning. To have this faith which is there, even though things may seem gloomy, is to have something special in your life which also has incredible therapeutic benefits.

**Heavy emotional burdens**

### Logotherapy

The founder of logotherapy (logos means sense), Victor E. Frankl, developed his theory during his long years of suffering in a concentration camp. Since then, he and his pupils have been able to help many people, who were in an apparently hopeless situation, to take courage, redefine the purpose of their lives and so find fulfilment and satisfaction.

The principles of logotherapy are that rather than resigning yourself to the things in your life that are bad or making you unhappy, you can change your way of thinking which will help you get a better grip on your life.

## Meditation

This is another method of achieving mental stabilization that shouldn't be underestimated. You may think that this type of system, with its connotations of the Far East and its associations with gurus and asceticism, hasn't got much to teach an enlightened European.

Yet, it is a method long known in both East and West for attaining greater serenity and mental harmony by making an 'inward journey'. This kind of regular exercise in submerging the self, switching off external stimuli while the consciousness remains wakeful, has a whole range of positive effects. These have been clearly demonstrated through the experience of many meditators worldwide and by scientific research, particularly in the USA.

**Serenity and mental harmony**

**Getting a better grip on life**

The benefits of meditation include enhanced physical and mental well-being, increased creativity, expanded wealth of imagination, improved sleep, a greater capacity to concentrate, richer creativity, more self-assurance, sounder judgement, and a reduction in feelings of anxiety and depressive moods. An easing of chronic illnesses such as asthma, eczema, migraine or addictions is frequently reported.

**Important**

It is important that you are introduced to meditation by a trained specialist, so that you don't form bad habits that could have adverse effects.

The most widely available training is provided at the training centres of Transcendental Meditation (TM). The basic course teaches you about meditation techniques.

The procedure is simple: you sit down in a comfortable position and mentally repeat over and over again the word selected by the meditation instructor. In itself this has no meaning but takes effect entirely from its soothing sound (though you only 'hear' it mentally and don't speak it). Even children can do this, from the age of four onwards.

You should find that you reach a relaxed state quite quickly. This will give you a feeling of detachment that can't be compared with either the sleeping or the waking state. This state of consciousness has a lasting effect which you will find helps with mental harmonization.

**Perform meditation regularly**

The important thing is to perform meditation regularly, for 20 minutes (and no more) twice a day – preferably in the morning and late afternoon or early evening. Anyone who has been convinced of the success of this method will gladly give up such a relatively modest space of time.

### Autogenic training

Developed by German psychiatrist, Johannes Schultz, in the 1930s, this is a combination of western methods of auto-suggestion and some ancient yoga techniques.

Autogenic training consists of six basic exercises aimed at inducing profound and healing relaxation. These exercises are carried out while the mind is concentrated on various physical states, for example feelings of heaviness ('my right arm is heavy'), feelings of warmth ('my left leg is warm'), a coolness of the brow, calming the breathing. Each instruction is visualized and repeated three times. Autogenic training is taught in hospitals and private clinics by psychologists, psychiatrists and, occasionally, in adult education classes.

### The Silva method

This therapy was was developed in 1966 by José Silva, a Mexican American. It is a form of dynamic meditation which, by consciously taking control of the mind, can control stress and tension. The Silva technique aims to put people in touch with the deeper and more creative levels of their minds. Deep relaxation is reached by counting backwards from ten to one.

**Dynamic meditation**

Other techniques practised include positive thinking ('negative thoughts don't affect me') and visualization. The latter means picturing as vividly as possibly the thing that you want most in life and what you would like to achieve.

No limitations are imposed on your own fantasy, whether it is a new car, a dream job or the man or woman of your life. And you also picture yourself as you would like to be – attractive, nimble, cheerful, slim, healthy, vital.

The method is based on the theory that thoughts are a form of mobile energy and we create our reality by what we think. Someone who thinks of nothing but illness will end up falling sick (or not getting better); someone who believes **Belief** in his own eventual success or healing with unshakable certainty, as though it were already a reality, will be granted it. Belief can move mountains, as we know from the Bible – but generally too little use is made of this knowledge.

## The powerhouse of the subconscious

All these techniques, which contribute to our mental harmonization and physical health, operate by means of our 'subconscious powerhouse'. With the current bias towards **Sixth sense** scientific reasoning, it is easy to lose sight of this important centre, which is responsible for our 'sixth sense' – our intuition and our creative powers. This is the part of us that often instinctively makes the right decisions and produces better ideas for solving our problems than logic or reason.

**The profound effect of using cassettes:** modern technology provides us with a convenient means of programming and activating the deep layers of our mental condition. There are many relaxation tapes that operate directly on our subconscious, helping us achieve greater concentration, sounder sleep and freedom from stress, anxiety and depression.

Sometimes only relaxing and calming music can be **Relaxation** heard. Through a technical process the spoken words are **tapes** made inaudible, but they are still picked up by our subconscious nevertheless.

These subliminal cassettes have already been amazingly successful in cases of sleeplessness. Another side benefit is the elimination of the need for sleeping pills and the damaging effects they can have.

## Alcohol – an addictive substance

Habituation to an addictive substance is often the reason for people always feeling slightly unwell. This applies to the consumption of alcohol, which is now not only socially acceptable but has actually become a part of our way of life. Beer at mealtimes, or in the local pub, wine with food or while watching TV, drinks of all kinds at parties, whisky for a nightcap – these are as much a part of our everyday life as our daily bread.

But very few of us face up to the fact that with every glass of alcohol we give the brain a small dose of poison, not to speak of its effect on the liver and the heart. For a long time the body seems to tolerate even a continuous supply of this intoxicant; more than that, it leads us to believe we are doing it some good in this way.

We actually feel more relaxed and cheerful when we have had a drink and we fail to realize that this euphoriant effect is itself a typical symptom of poisoning. Most people don't make the connection between the regular consumption of alcohol and nervousness, irritability, restless sleep, lack of concentration, aggression, lack of drive, depression and putting on weight. Quite the reverse, and this is where our body plays the next trick on us. Since alcohol breeds dependency, we start to feel something is lacking if we drink apple juice instead of alcohol. Often it isn't until we have had an alcoholic drink that we feel noticably more lively and confident.

Although there is nothing wrong with enjoying the occasional drink with a meal, or when on holiday, it is when drinking becomes a habit that it becomes the main cause of a variety of health problems and indispositions. In more extreme cases people move beyond drinking as a social habit on to the path towards alcoholism.

Food-allergy sufferers, however, should impose a strict prohibition on themselves, and they should also remember that they could also react to the basic materials or other ingredients from which drinks are made, such as the wheat and yeast in some beers, the grain in whisky, and the grapes or sulphur in wine.

If you do decide to change your lifestyle and start to take more care of your body, you need to remember that people are, in general, creatures of habit. This means that it is often difficult for us to replace a bad habit with a good one so that any permanent changes will take time and perseverance.

It is best to try to make one change at a time rather than

suddenly turning your whole life inside-out. If you try to achieve too much in one go you could find it becomes overwhelming and that all your good resolutions will disappear leaving you back where you started.

It is also important too make allowances for yourself. If you find yourself slipping back into your old habits, don't be despondent, just renew your resolution to lead a healthy life and try again. With perseverance you will find eventually that a leading healthy way of life has become second nature to you.

### We have to take the initiative ourselves

Finally, when looking at allergies, we cannot ignore the extent to which our environmental conditions are to blame for their development.

Environmental poisons, to which we are all exposed nowadays, weaken the immune system and a weakened immune system opens the door to allergies. This applies in particular to people who, because of their genes, already suffer a natural disadvantage in this respect.

It is an open secret that because of the reckless way people deal with the environment, we are well on the way to destroying the basis for our existence.

Intensive farming and artificial fertilizers have ruined the soil and polluted the ground water with chemicals. Lakes and rivers are choked with poisons, the forests are diseased, the air we breathe is charged with contaminants, our food is refined and 'improved' – and we are all being asked to foot the bill.

Only by changing our own behaviour and making sacrifices in our private lives, by rejecting self-destructive luxury and thus setting a good example to our family, neighbours, friends and colleagues, will we be able to avoid the further destruction of the environment.

We need to use our power as consumers to get industry to change its ways. We should make it clear to our government that it can depend on our support if, without fearing a loss of votes at the next election, it has the courage to pass laws that really bite. Only if we support our environmental organizations by joining them will they be able to represent our interests effectively.

After all, who better to shake others out of their ignorance and apathy than people who have already been forced to recognize in their own bodies – through allergies – the consequences of environmental pollution?

# Useful addresses

The Faculty of Homeopathy
The Royal London
Homeopathic Hospital
Great Ormond Street
London WC1N 3HR
Tel: 0171 837 8833

The Hyperactive Children's
Support Group
71 Whyke Lake
Chichester
West Sussex PO19 2LD
Tel: 01903 725182
(10am – 1pm Tue-Fri)

The British Society for
Allergy and
Environmental Medicine
Acorns
Romsey Road
Cadnam
Southampton SO4 2NN
Tel: 01703 812124

British Society of Dowsers
Sycamore Cottage
Tamley Lane
Hasingleigh
Ashford
Kent TN25 5HW
Tel: 01233 75253

The Society of Homeopaths
2 Artizan Road
Northampton NN1 4HU
Tel: 01604 21400

The Chinese Medical Centre
Manvers Chambers
Manvers Street
Bath
Avon BA1 1PE
Tel: 01225 483393

Published originally under the title "Allergien – natürlich behandeln"
by Gräfe und Unzer Verlag GmbH, Munich
© 1992 Dr Sigrid Flade, D-83700 Rottach-Weissach

Authorized English language edition published by
Time-Life Books BV, 1066 Amsterdam
© 1996 Time-Life Books BV
First English language printing 1996

English translation by Carmona UK
Editorial Manager: Christine Noble
Editor: Alison Mackonochie
Layout/DTP: Dawn M<sup>C</sup>Ginn

ISBN 0 7054 3541 5

20 19 18 17 16 15 14 13 12 11 10 9 8 7 6 5 4 3 2 1